**PERSONAL TRAINER**
YOGA FOR LIFE

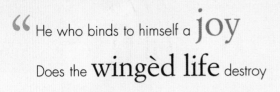

"He who binds to himself a joy

Does the **wingèd life** destroy

But he who kisses the joy as it flies

Lives in eternity's sunrise." WILLIAM BLAKE

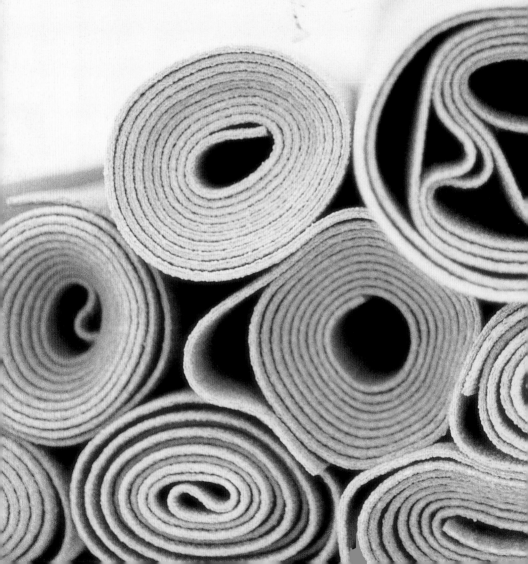

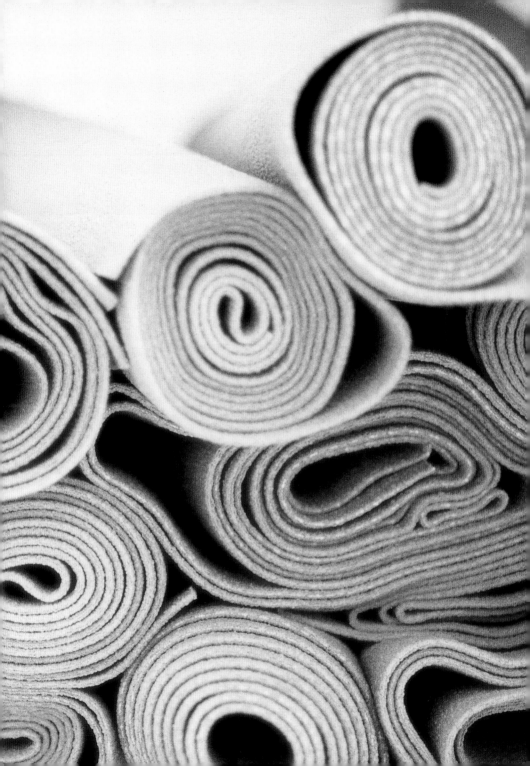

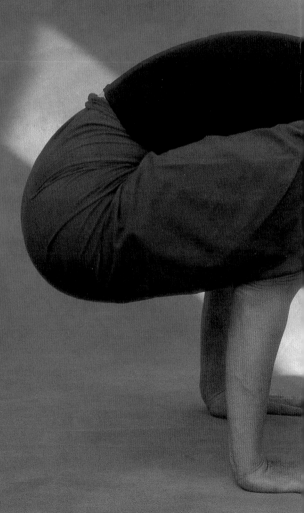

THIS IS A CARLTON BOOK

Design copyright © 2001 Carlton Books Limited
Text copyright © 2001 Liz Lark
Photographs copyright © Clare Park

This paperback edition published in 2010
by Carlton Books Limited
20 Mortimer Street
London
W1T 3JW

10 9 8 7 6 5 4 3 2 1

A CIP catalogue record for this book is available
from the British Library.

ISBN 978 1 84732 669 0

Printed in China

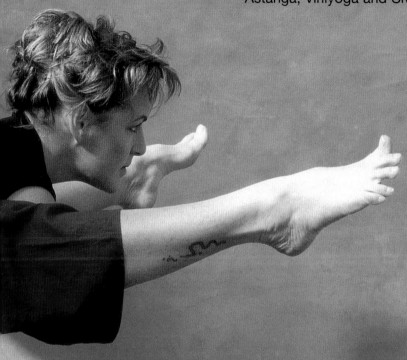

# PERSONAL TRAINER
## YOGA FOR LIFE
The at-home introduction to Iyengar,
Astanga, Viniyoga and Sivananda

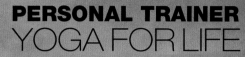

LIZ LARK

Photography by Clare Park

**CARLTON**

" Yoga is not [attained] through the Lotus posture and not by gazing at the **tip of the nose**.

Yoga, say the experts of yoga, is the

identity of the psyche

with the [transcendental] self. "

KULA ARNAVA TANTRA, TANTRIC TEXT

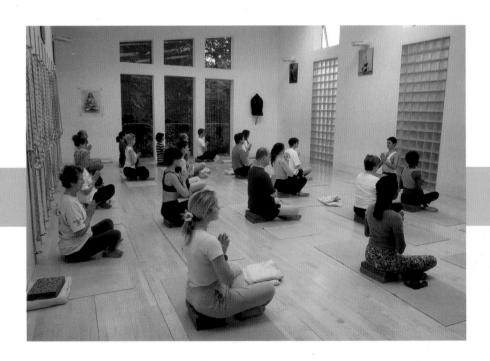

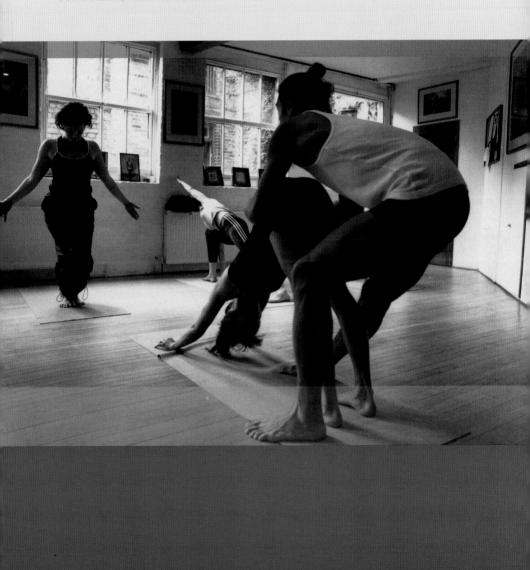

**"** The fabled musk deer searches the whole world over for the source of the scent that comes from within. **"** RAMAKRISHNA PARAMHAMSA, BIHAR SCHOOL OF YOGA

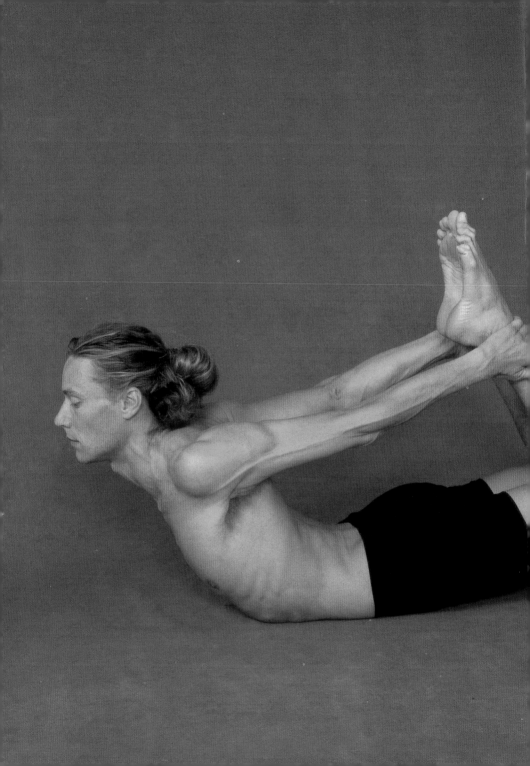

# CONTENTS

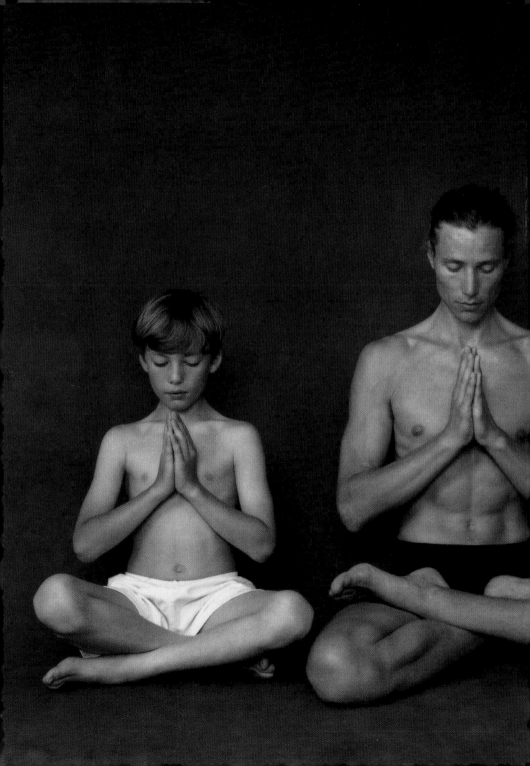

# CUTTING THROUGH THE CHAOS

" ...yoga is like a river that has been flowing for so many years. It has now entered the Western world. It will have many tributaries, it will swell. Our ancient people did a lot of research within themselves... One of the greatest gifts that yoga gives is observation; observation of the self and of others... Nothing is constant. Even science believes things will change. " T. K. V. DESIKACHAR, "THE ROLE OF YOGA IN THE NEXT MILLENNIUM", CONFERENCE, NARBONNE, FRANCE, 1999.

Yoga is a vast subject, a deep practice rooted in the mists of prehistory and developed by ancient seers who learned from nature and self-observation. Yoga encompasses many different approaches, styles and practices, but all the yogas share the same focus, namely transcendence, unity, oneness, bliss. Integral to all of them is the essence of the original Sanskrit word "yoga" meaning "union". In the practice of yoga, body is linked with mind, breath with movement, to bring about a feeling of balance, relaxation and wellbeing.

The yogic concept of fitness involves balancing and integrating all aspects of ourselves, and of our lives, which leads us towards inhabiting our bodies and becoming comfortable with ourselves. This is a continual, developing process, a journey from agony to ecstasy. (The Greek "ekstasis" means to "stand outside" the ordinary self.) Yoga offers us a way of observing the drama of our lives with detachment, a way of seeing with greater clarity, motivated by what yoga academic Georg Feuerstein describes as the "impulse towards transcendence". In order to dwell in the sublime, the place he describes as the "timeless quintessence of all beings and things", we must train body and mind, focusing attention like a laser beam in order to transcend our conditioning. In yoga, we learn how to observe, not how to judge. We learn to surrender, let go and thus suffer less.

Feuerstein observed that the greatness of the West lies in its control of the outer world and the greatness of the East lies in its control of the unseen inner world. India's "sacred technicians" have been developing this unseen inner world for millennia. Father Bede Griffiths, a Benedictine monk and Abbot of Prinknash Abbey, Gloucester, left England to spend most of his life in India as a sannyassin (wandering renunciate). He suggested that the root cause of the failure of modern civilization is that it has lost connection with "the centre, the ground of reality and truth", and that the only way to recover this is through a complete turnaround ("metanoia"); a surrender and return to a source of truth.

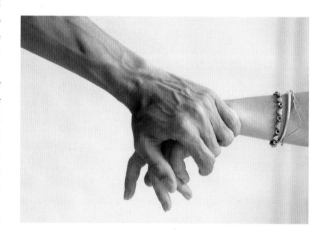

Despite the external success of the West, Colin Norman, editor of *Science* magazine, has described material technology as "the god that limps". This is a reference to the Greek god of blacksmiths, the ironworking Hephaestos, the first child of Zeus and Hera who was thrown out of heaven because he was born ugly.

66 Know **thyself**, and thou shalt know the universe. 99 ANCIENT GREEKS

# Benefits of yoga

The Bihar School of Yoga in Mungar, India, describes yoga as a healing system that can be used to treat many ailments and mental disorders. All yoga systems, both Western and Eastern methods, are part of a broad spectrum of healing; deep healing, from the core takes time as opposed to quick fixes like adding sticking plaster to a wound, takes time, so it is important to be patient.

Yoga tackles imbalance and disease by:
- massaging the internal organs
- toning the nerves
- improving respiration, energy and vitality
- purifying the body internally
- relaxing the mind and removing anxieties
- encouraging positive thoughts and self-acceptance.

Swami Pragyamurti, Satyananda yoga teacher (see Chapter 4), believes the benefits of yoga are wide-ranging, from the abstract to the concrete. She outlines three areas: firstly, improved physical health; secondly, relaxation in body and mind through pranayama (breathing practices) and meditation; thirdly, the benefit of "going within" oneself, which brings peace and restoration. Yoga enables us to "live as we want to, usefully, lovingly and interestingly", bringing discipline, focus and personal integrity. It empowers and transforms, as we begin to "own" ourselves.

# Origins

In India there is no word for religion, only "dharma", which translates as "right being". India has spawned four major spiritual traditions: Hinduism, Buddhism, Sikhism and Jainism, an ascetic religion close to Buddhism. The dominant religion is Hinduism, which refers to the entire culture of the inhabitants of India and to the traditions which link it to the ancient Vedic culture of 6000 years ago. Hinduism inhabits a world of myth, and its plethora of gods are symbols of divine mystery. Yoga has emerged from this, but is practised by people of all ideologies and cultures.

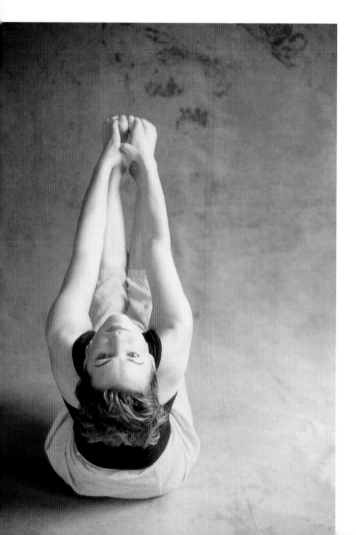

### Vedanta – from separation to synthesis

The *Veda*, the earliest sacred literature of India, contain the first references to yoga. Written in Sanskrit, the mother of many Indo-european languages, in 1500 BCE, from these taproots grew the *Upanishads*, about 800 years later, which give teachings on meditation. According to Vedic philosophy, the individual self is alienated from its transcendent self, and this isolation is the root cause of human suffering.

Vedanta recognizes that looking outside ourselves for wholeness brings disappointment and pain, and as long as our male and female energies remain unbalanced, we remain desperate for the company of others to ease this indeterminate ache. The Buddhist Tantric monk, Lama Yeshe, suggests that all the problems of the world can be traced to this nameless ache, a feeling of not being whole, of being lonely as opposed to alone or "all-one".

Known as the eternal culture, Vedanta imparts the message of "oneness", a philosophy offering a universal principle that unites all, dissolving barriers of difference and separation.

> " Kill with the sword of wisdom the doubt born of ignorance that lies in thy heart... Be a warrior and kill desire, the powerful enemy of the soul. "
>
> THE BHAGAVAD GITA

## The Sutra

"Sutra" means literally "thread" and the Sutra are defined as threads of wisdom. Patanjali, who is thought to have lived at the beginning of the first (Christian) millennium, crystallized the teachings of the Yoga Sutra into Eight Limbs (see page 17). Yoga does not conflict with other religions because the Sutra do not tell you to follow a particular path and can support people of all belief systems.

# Professor T. Krishnamacharya

Professor T. Krishnamacharya was a twentieth-century "acharya", that is one who has travelled far on the journey and lived what he taught, and he is responsible for much of the yoga currently taught in the West.

Born in Karnataka, India, Krishnamacharya's ancestors practised yoga as long ago as AD 800. He studied first with his father, then formally at various universities, where he attained high levels of academic achievement learning the principles of Ayurveda, classical natural Indian medicine. A renowned Sanskrit scholar, he was fluent in the ancient language from an early age, one of the few in the country who could speak it.

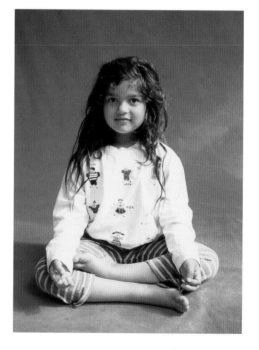

Krishnamacharya found his spiritual teacher, Sri Ramamohan Brahmachari, in the Tibetan Himalayas near Mount Kailash, staying with him for eight years. Brahmachari was a "householder", that is he lived a family life, and he told Krishnamacharya to teach yoga in the city, living among the people, as opposed to following the monastic tradition of other schools.

In 1931, the Maharaja of Mysore, a student of Krishnamacharya, invited him to open a yoga school in the Jagan Palace. This became the rigorous training ground that spawned the teaching methods of B. K. S. Iyengar, T. K. V. Desikachar and Sri K. Pattabhi Jois, all of whom followed the householder tradition. Desikachar, Krishnamacharya's son, studied daily with him developing the strand of Viniyoga (Chapter 1); Iyengar became master of alignment and depth of asana (Chapter 2); and Pattabhi Jois became master teacher of Astanga Vinyasa (Chapter 3).

Despite his learning, teaching and dedication, Krishnamacharya refused to allow anyone to call him a guru, or even a yogi, only an "acharya". He died aged 100. Krishnamacharya considered Patanjali's Yoga Sutra to be the key text for guidance and with Desikachar he synthesized a vast body of yogic and religious understanding. The aim of his life was to disseminate yoga among as many people as possible and he believed in adapting the practice of yoga to suit the individual's needs.

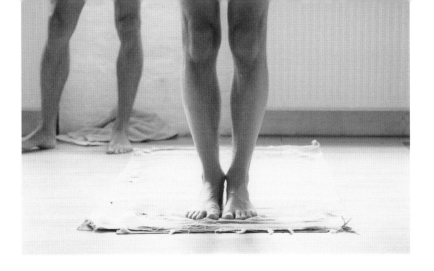

# The Eight Limb system

This is the system of yoga crystallized by the sage Patanjali. These Eight Limbs
("ast-angas") are integral to all the yogas in varying degrees.

**1.** Yama: restraints, rules of conduct

    ahimsa: non-violence, the supreme restraint – yoga for life!

    satya: truthfulness

    asteya: non-stealing

    brahmacharya: continence, self-control

    aparigraha: non-grasping

**2.** Niyama: discipline of the body and mind, observances

    saucha: inner and outer cleanliness, aspiring to sattva guna (see page 37)

    santosha: contentment

    tapas: discipline, practice

    svadhyaya: spiritual study

    Iswarapranidhana: surrender to the highest principle

**3.** Asana: steady posture, poise, balance

**4.** Pranayama: breathing practices, literally control of the vital force

**5.** Pratyahara: withdrawal of the senses

**6.** Dharana: mind focus, concentration

**7.** Dhyana: meditation

**8.** Samadhi: absorption through meditation, bliss, piercing the veil
    of "maya" (illusion)

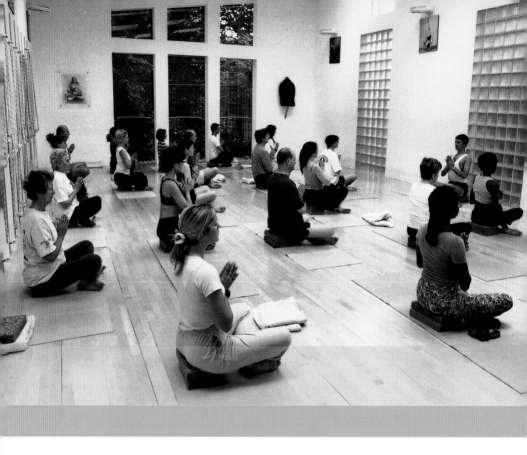

When we do yoga, we give space for our system to unite with the self, something more subtle than the mind, which tells us what to do. Suffering makes us look for the key to the door, to go in. We need some help to enter the door where we are centred... this has to be done very carefully. When we are there, centred, we have nothing to be afraid of. "

T. K. V. DESIKACHAR, SPEAKING OF THE JOURNEY FROM THE EXTERNAL TO THE INTERNAL

# Finding the key

Like Alice travelling through the looking glass to a different reality, with yoga we can see things with greater clarity. Yoga gives us keys to the doors of change, but it's up to us to choose which ones to use. To open the front door of this mysterious and beautiful castle we need to find the key that suits us best. In the methods of Hatha yoga the first keys to unlocking the body are asana, breathing and other preparations for meditation.

## Hatha yoga

Each form of yoga is an enormous subject in itself (further reading suggestions are given on pages 152–3). The form best known in the West is Hatha, meaning literally "force" and symbolically the union of the sun and moon. Hatha yoga is an umbrella term for yogas that employ physical and breathing exercises to still the mind, enabling us to transcend its conditioning. Thus the two most commonly used Limbs of Hatha yoga are asana (body posture, the Third Limb) and pranayama (breathing practice, the Fourth Limb). Pattabhi Jois says that practising posture and breathing can gradually help us practise the First and Second Limbs, restraints not by force or dogma but through experience and choice.

The first four chapters of this book concentrate on four Hatha methods practised in the West: Viniyoga, Iyengar, Astanga Vinyasa and Sivananda. Traditional aspects of yoga also include:

- Raja yoga, the "royal path ", shares the Hatha aim of mastering oneself
- Jnana (knowledge), yoga of self-enquiry through study
- Bhakti (heart), yoga of devotion
- Karma (action), yoga of unconditional service (a central concept of the Bhagavad Gita, see page 122)
- Tantra

The mother system of Hatha yoga, Tantra (Chapter 5) is said to have begun when woman took her first breath. Its origins are shrouded in mystery and it encompasses a vast cradle of practices, one of which is yoga. Tantra is the science of expanding and liberating consciousness to gain knowledge. It is concerned with the marriage of masculine and feminine energy, synthesizing the material and spiritual realms, to attain ecstasy or bliss. It worships the feminine psychic principle, represented by Shakti. The goal of yoga is for our latent, psychic energy (symbolized by kundalini, a coiled snake) to be released

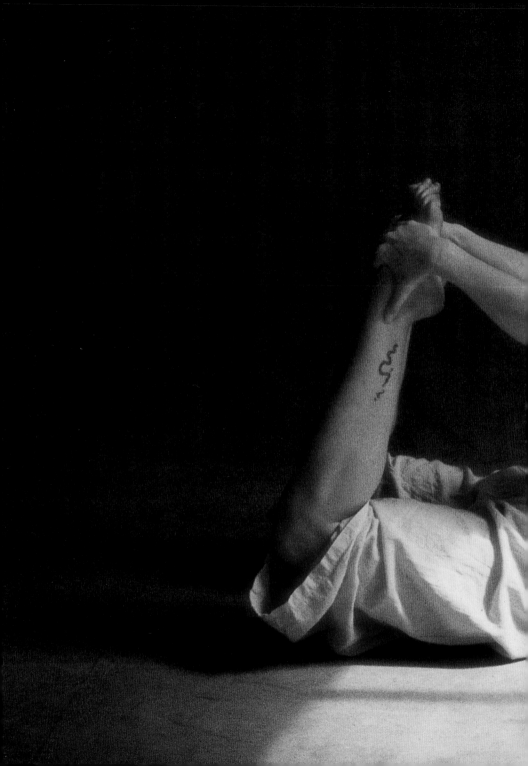

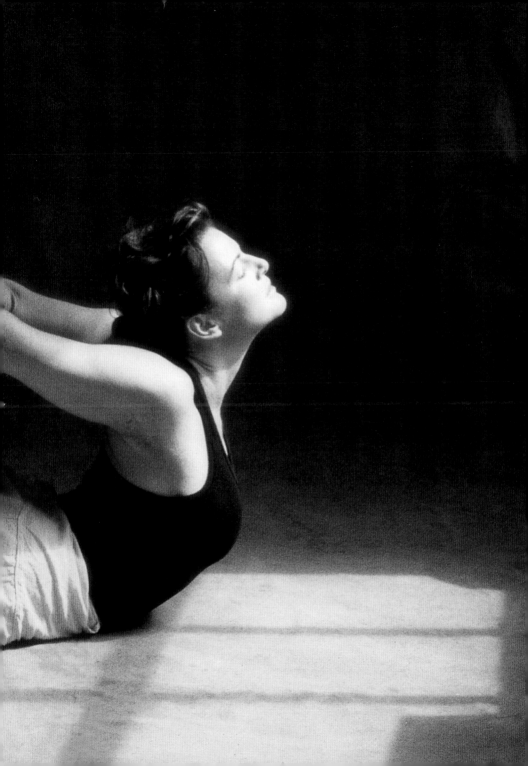

through the union of Shakti with her spouse Shiva. In this awakening, lower grades of energy are absorbed into higher grades through the "subtle body".

Tantra practice includes the use of symbolic sounds (mantras) and visual patterns (yantras and mandalas) for meditation.

## Buddhist Tantra – breaking the cycle of pain

Buddhist Tantra has flourished in Tibet for more than 1000 years and can be traced back 2500 years to the time of Buddha himself. It asserts that every human being has the potential within to transform experiences into happiness and bliss, by harnessing all aspects of our human energy, especially the energy of our desires.

Normally our desires bring us dissatisfaction and further craving, but if used skilfully they can be our most precious source of spiritual fulfilment and, with dedicated practice, we can harness our inner potential.

Tantra recognizes that we yearn to be happy and this desire drives all our actions. However, this grasping for pleasure keeps us swimming in an ocean of "samsara" (to circle) where we suffer a perpetual cycle of frustrations. Buddhism acknowledges that attachment leads to pain, but the denial or suppression of pleasure, and the guilt that surrounds it, is yet another form of grasping, locking us into a limited view of ourselves.

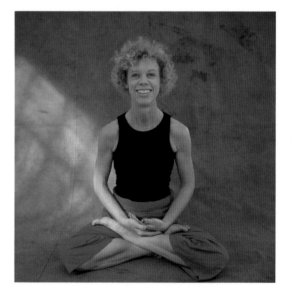

Tantra accepts the Vedic philosophy that we must strive to unite the male and female energies within us to break the cycle of pain.

"From my practice I get real joy. Pranayama lets your inner light shine from your eyes."

Catriona has practised yoga for more than 20 years, endlessly fascinated to learn about different styles and aspects and ultimately finding that they all work with the same fundamentals: tuning into the potential of your natural body energy.

"It's a lifetime process of self-discovery. It's not just an excuse to cut yourself off from things, but to become more comfortable in the world, which is what 'asana' means: comfortable posture."

# Tools of yoga

Hatha yoga provides tangible methods and techniques rooted in physicality which mould the body and mind, and enable us to work through the emotional layers of ourselves to uncover our spirituality. The processes teach us to nurture the inner life so often stifled in our chaotic world.

## Asana

Asana, body postures, cleanse and tone the body from the inside out, massaging internal organs and realigning and strengthening the spine. By realigning the body and balancing the left and right sides we avoid injury and damaging imbalance. Asana also soothe the mind, bringing it home to a calm place. The mind gradually becomes liberated from the conditioned patterns of thinking ("samskara") which bind it, and begins a journey from the head to the heart, as the practice teaches us to surrender. This is healing mentally and physically. Swami Pragyamurti explains that yoga has to be experienced to be understood properly, and you must be open, courageous and humorous enough to keep going.

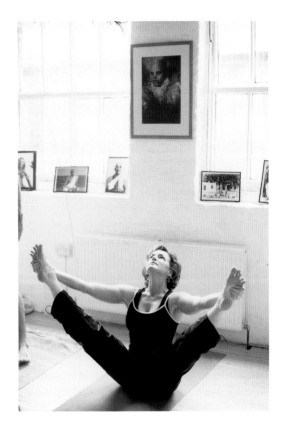

*Combine **intellectual knowledge** with the willingness to experience. Know it from the* **depths** *of your own being.*

SWAMI PRAGYAMURTI

## Drishti

Drishti means gaze points. There are nine gaze points in yoga that help to deepen concentration during asanas (see Chapter 3).

## Suryanamaskara

Suryanamaskara are sun salutations consisting of a sequence of 12 positions, traditionally practised at dawn 12 times – once for each month of the year. Their origins probably predate yoga.

## Mudras

Mudras, meaning "to delight in", a feature of Tantra practice, are symbolic hand gestures that concentrate and channel energy flow in the body.

## Pranayama

Pranayama is the control of the vital and psychic energy in the body through breathing practices (from "prana" meaning cosmic energy, creative life force – invisible but of the utmost importance). Pranayama soothes and restores us, removing anxieties and fear.

## Ujjayi

Ujjayi is deep thoracic breathing, i.e. from the ribcage, that calms the whole system. It is achieved with a jalandhara bandha (see below) and makes you feel as if your breath is moving from the throat down to the heart with a cave-like resonance.

## Bandhas

These are energy support locks or seals, and they help to awaken and direct the creative energy in the body and aid pranayama. Osteopath Mary O'Leary explains that bandha control helps to strengthen the abdominal muscles, which engage the lower back muscles, thus strengthening the rest of the back. Traditionally, the spiritual aspirant was introduced to bandhas secretly after mastering complex asanas. The bandhas we are dealing with are:

- Jalandhara – restraint of the jugular notch. The glottis at the back of the throat is narrowed and the chin is tucked in towards the chest. The breath is thus stretched and controlled.

- Uddiyana – the "flying up lock" which is said to harness the mind. The lower abdominal organs are drawn inwards and upwards, pulling the lower abdomen from the pubic bone to the navel towards the spine. A feeling of lightness is cultivated. This tones the belly, reduces fat in the stomach, massages the intestines and thus reduces constipation.

- Mula bandha – rather than a physical lock, mula bandha is a pranic, energetic technique, involving the contraction of the perineum, the section of the pelvic floor between the anus and genitals – for women the cervix, for men the root of the penis. This improves sexual control and the health of the pelvic region.

" Uddiyana is a **blessing** to humanity. It imparts beautiful health, strength, vigour and vitality to the practitioner. "

SWAMI SIVANANDA

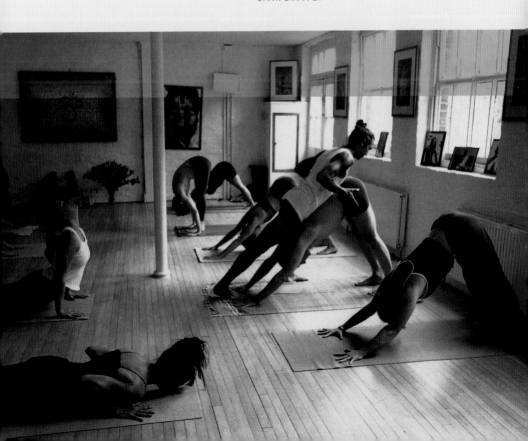

## Relaxation

Relaxation practices, including "yoga nidra" (yogic sleep), remove anxieties and mental anguish, as well as physiologically allowing the body to restore itself. Savasana, the Corpse posture, is a helpful relaxation position with which to close a yoga session.

## Meditation

Concentration on a mantra, a flower or anything else you choose develops "single-pointedness" which leads into meditation, enabling us to step into the moment, leaving anxieties behind.

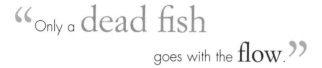

"Only a dead fish goes with the flow."

There is a misconception that being in the moment, i.e. going with the flow, means denying all responsibilities, when in fact it involves harnessing all of ourselves, facing our fears, focusing and envisioning our future, and only then letting go! Being in the moment is a serious business requiring tremendous attention without tension, drawing the mind to a single focus and cutting through the chaos – this is yoga.

Pilates teacher and yoga practitioner Muriel Carrasco says:
"Yoga, particularly Astanga and Iyengar, encourages proper body use and body awareness. It teaches you the real body–mind connection through the breath. There's nothing magic about it: it's a science, it's pragmatic. The yamas [First Limb] are not limiting. The morals are about freeing yourself. For example, not lying makes you brave. Self-discipline leads to freedom."

Pilates is a form of body conditioning that trains specific muscle groups thoroughly and cultivates proper body use. Pilates techniques go well with yoga. The bandha control and deep diaphragmatic breathing with vinyasa movements bring concentration. The specific movements of pilates enhance body awareness and feed very well into yoga practice, as do the elements of alignment and subtle release of the Alexander Technique.

# The key methods

### Viniyoga

Viniyoga was developed by the master teacher Professor. T. Krishnamacharya and is now continued by his son T. K. V. Desikachar. An individual and pro-gressive system, Viniyoga is gradual and gentle . Although some group class-es are taught, traditionally the yoga was passed on one-to-one and personal tuition is favoured. There is no set course; a programme is tailored to suit each student's needs.

Viniyoga practice flows with soft ujjayi (deep breathing) that lasts longer than the duration of the asana stretch. Viniyoga is accessible to everyone and is excellent for all stages of life. It can also be applied therapeutically.

### Iyengar yoga

A student of Krishnamacharya, B. K. S. Iyengar is an architect of the body. His study of yoga focuses on mastery of alignment and precision of posture to a fantastic level: "The yogi uses his body to refine his inner intelligence."

A technically correct style, with strong foundation principles, Iyengar yoga is a rigorous, thorough training in body and mind, which teaches us to access and wake up every cell of the body so that "every fibre is singing!"

With excellent use of props and modifications, Iyengar yoga is particularly suitable for specific needs, older people and those with injuries. Specialist classes can be designed to suit all needs and abilities, and can include remedial work.

### Astanga Vinyasa yoga

This is a dynamic, exhilarating dance of yoga, the master teacher of which is Sri K. Pattabhi Jois. It has a dramatic effect on the shape and tone of the body if regularly practised, and sheds toxins, fat and stress quickly. Although immediately appealing to young, fit people, this challenging, warrior yoga, if properly taught, is accessible to anyone who can walk.

The foundation sequence begins with standing sun saluta-tions. Asanas are linked to a focused breath and the practice is constantly flowing. Derek Ireland, who helped spread Astanga in Europe, called this "no bullshit yoga"! The practice is expe-riential and philosophy is little talked about during a session.

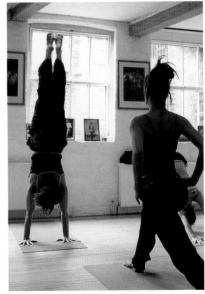

### Sivananda yoga

Named after Swami Sivananda, a karma yogi from southern India, this holistic, rounded yoga has spawned many off-shoots in the West, including Satyananda yoga, to be discussed in Chapter 4. Sivananda yoga embraces all yoga paths, including karma, bhakti and jnana. It is an integral system based on five principles: proper exercise, proper breathing, proper relaxation, proper diet and positive thinking/meditation. Alignment training is not of central importance. This type of yoga is accessible to everyone, all ages and body types.

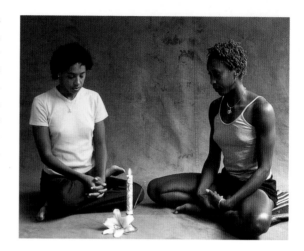

# Choosing the right method

The methods demonstrated in this book will present the main elements of yoga, which can be applied to other forms as well. The aim is to enable you to find a method that suits your lifestyle and body type (see page 37), so, rather than adapting yoga to fit your life, eventually, imperceptibly, it floods all aspects of your existence. By learning key facets of the main methods and practising the sessions illustrated you can establish which method may suit you best. Then go and find a class.

As we move through life it is a question of practising the yoga that balances us. As we change and adapt, so will the yoga practice. Each yoga method has the same ingredients, but in slightly different quantities. For example, every Viniyoga and Sivananda class includes pranayama, but in Viniyoga it comes at the end of posture work and in the Sivananda system breathing practices come at the beginning of the session. The Iyengar system places tremendous emphasis on the precision of alignment in asana (postures), and pranayama is reserved for a later stage, once the student is accomplished in asana. In Astanga Vinyasa, breathing and postures are synthesized right from the start and are inseparable, but other pranayama practices are not taught until one has a strong, steady asana practice.

It is important to approach yoga with an open mind; each form may enrich your life.

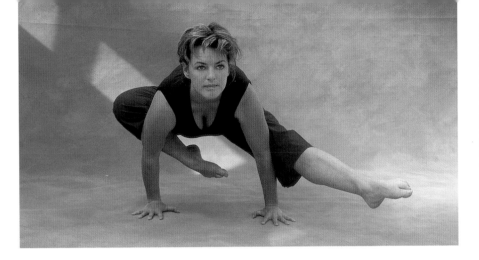

# Yoga for specific groups

### Beginners

Try any style that attracts. Iyengar provides a superb introduction for alignment awareness; Sivananda gives a gentle introduction, offers a clearly defined
"yoga lifestyle", and does not emphasize alignment awareness; Viniyoga's personal, nurturing approach is profound on every level; and the challenge and
physicality of Astanga will suit certain personalities. Each style will be con-
veyed in its own way by different teachers, so explore!

### Children

Yoga is fantastic for kids. It needs to be fun, creative and constant. Yoga keeps
our spines free and lithe, and maintains flexibility, so start early. Many poses
are named after animals and nature, so they appeal visually to children and
learning them stimulates their imagination. It can also help children to relax.
"It kind of makes you all droopy, like when I'm sleepy," says Dominic, who
practises his own relaxation technique in the dentist's chair, taking a huge sigh
to release tension, much to the dentist's surprise!

" In my view, it is not useful to think of different styles of yoga: this is

simply yoga, which comes from a vast and ancient source. The only authentic

yoga is one which works for each person according to circumstances

and needs, and there are many possibilities. " DESIKACHAR, THE HEART OF YOGA

Advanced poses, such as headstands, should not be taught until the age of 14, when growth slows down, since they can interfere with hormones and bone formation.

No specific style is recommended although jumping and dynamic Vinyasa works well because most kids are like jumping beans! Krishnamacharya taught this system to children, keeping their attention in a constant, flowing sequence, with challenging asanas. Astanga Vinyasa is recommended after puberty, not before when bones are still forming.

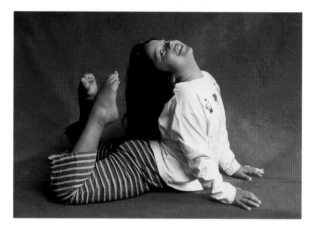

Children have the advantage of having less fear and prejudice than adults. Iyengar teaches classes of 60 to 70 children. He comments: "Children love to have variations, freshness. We have to see they don't get bored. They are not afraid, they are strong. They need speed, strength and variety," adding that at first they have to be treated on the physical level, then at 16 or 17 they can learn about the mind, and later about self. When B. K. S. Iyengar, Sri K. Pattabhi Jois and T. K. V. Desikachar were young students of Professor Krishnamacharya, photographs demonstrate that their training was indeed intense and gymnastic.

### The elderly

Soft, gentle Sivananda and the personal approach of Viniyoga are ideal for older folk whereas stimulating Iyengar and Astanga asanas wake up the body and mind, preventing the faculties from becoming sluggish! People of every age need stimulation: an alert mind keeps the body young. Yoga can be adapted to meet the needs of old and young alike.

66 Whether young, old or very old, sick or feeble, one can attain more powers through practice. 99

*HATHA YOGA PRADIPIKA*, OPENING CHAPTER

# Proprioception

Yoga awakens the body's intelligence through proprioception. Proprioceptors are sensory nerve endings in the body which are like little eyes receiving stimuli, keeping joints, muscles and tendons active , thus preventing injury.

Proprioception is the body's response to being slightly off balance and can be developed through balancing exercises such as standing on one leg, with one eye closed, catching a ball. Proprioceptive training runs through all the standing, balancing asanas for we are awakening every fibre in the body. When someone complains of having a weak ankle, it is not the ankle that is weak. The proprioceptors need activating around it to create support and thus it is essential that as we get older we keep these responses awake. When Iyengar talks about the difference between an "alert" and "dull" kneecap, he is talking about proprioception; the "intellectual eye" he refers to in the cells of the body is cultivating the body's ability to respond and restore balance through quick reflexes.

Professional footballers in rehab have been advised that the single most important thing that must be developed is proprioception to avoid further injury.

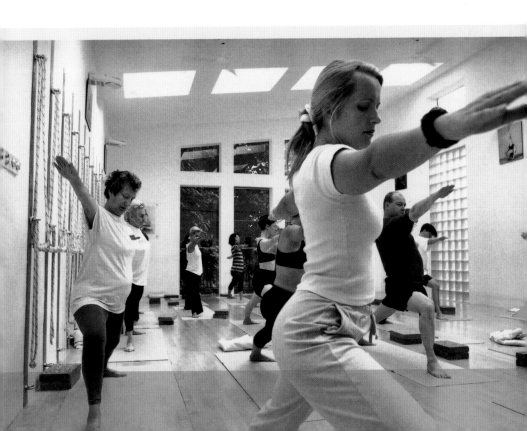

# Yoga for specific conditions

## Addiction

As even the midnight lemonade drinker knows, we cannot get rid of our addictions by hiding and suppressing them. Writer and teacher Justine Hardy says we have to be brave to do yoga and it is the greatest challenge we will ever undertake. We must practise with love for and acceptance of ourselves. The deep meditative work of the Bihar School and the Integral yoga of the British School of Yoga lead one gently on the journey into the mind. An experienced teacher is essential for this deep work if we are gradually to acknowledge the mind's tricks. We need to observe our conditioned patterns of thinking (samskaras) moment by moment to free ourselves from them.

Yoga can be useful in helping people to come off drugs, and a number of teachers have worked in detox programmes. Regular yoga practice helps people to think clearly about themselves. On alcohol, Swami Pragyamurti comments, "If they could only stop at the jolly stage!" On smoking, Swami Sivananda said, "When you want a cigarette, sit in Vajrasana [see page 70] and smoke with utmost awareness."

David Dunning-White, 43, has been practising Astanga yoga for a year, during recovery from drugs. Following his treatment with Alcoholics Anonymous he was "clean" for four years, but found he was still neurotic. He believes yoga has cured him:

"It has cured a large part of my neurosis. It realigns me ...I have become peaceful. It's extraordinary. I was walking through Knightsbridge, London, two days ago, and I felt completely still and whole and infinitely relaxed, in the middle of the Knightsbridge traffic... I was bigtime into hedonism, partying, drugs, because it took me into a different state of consciousness. But I was doing it the wrong way. Patanjali mentions drugs and herbs to open up the psychic centres... LSD takes you into the garden, but at six o'clock the gardener comes and chucks you out!! The proper paths of meditation take you through the main gate and the gardener doesn't chuck you out!"

" Ever since I was a kid I was fascinated by yoga. It was one of the only things that felt right for me. I lost myself in addiction, and I knew that yoga was the only way home. " BIBA LOGAN, SIVANANDA TEACHER

## Depression

Depression has been described as "the inability to find the way to feel who you are". Psychologist Carl Jung defined depression as dissociation and separation from the self, which causes alienation, isolation and lack of purpose. Yoga brings us back to the self, integrating all its facets and bringing union.

Sensitive, individual Viniyoga and soft Sivananda both employ breathing practices which soothe and restore, working subtly to clear away negativity. Breathing through mental pain brings about acceptance, another facet of yoga's meaning.

Astanga Vinyasa's endorphin releases can generate a change in awareness and cut through depression. This method can be extraordinarily healing and empowering. It helps to shed the negative patterns of thinking which imprison us. One teacher finds Astanga is particularly useful for people coming off antidepressants.

All the methods suggested here change how you feel if practised regularly – daily if possible. Search, and you will find the key! The hardest and the most important thing is to step on your mat and begin.

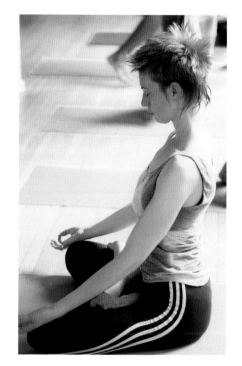

## Injury

A very soft practice is advisable when injured, and if that means remaining in Savasana, the Corpse posture, for your entire practice, so be it. Some injuries may make asana practice impossible and the higher Limbs of breathing, concentration and meditation may be more appropriate. It depends on the injury; you must listen to what the body needs. It may call for rest. If you are bedridden, you can lie in such a way that the heart is nourished with healthy blood, for yoga oxygenates the system and stimulates the organs with fresh blood. Pranayama, breathing practices, and bhakti, yoga of devotion achieved through contemplation or worship, are healing on a subtle, not just physical, level. Healing through yoga means reaching a state of grace and acceptance.

If the injury is muscular, it can be useful to work through it physically, although it can be painful. You must distinguish between "sweet" pain and pain which sets off alarm bells. Be sensitive and do not force the practice.

Iyengar yoga can include specialist remedial classes. B. K. S. Ivengar says that you can practise it with illness but not with a fever, when you should rest.

Richard Brown began Iyengar yoga at the age of 58, encouraged by a friend who recommended remedial yoga for his knee after a cartilage operation.

The body knows what is best. Ann Allen, practitioner of over 30 years, began yoga in her twenties to strengthen her legs when varicose veins developed after childbirth. Asked if you should practise when injured, she answers, "Most definitely. It cured injuries for me when nothing else helped."

It is important to discern what is appropriate according to the injury. In Viniyoga an individual programme will be prescribed. For dedicated practitioners, yoga is an ongoing relationship. As long as you can breathe, visualize and meditate, you can practice.

### Caution

If in any doubt, seek a specialist class. For example, if you have a history of disc injury, you must be extremely cautious in forward bends. To launch into an advanced Astanga Vinyasa practice could be foolish; you must start in a beginners' class and learn correct alignment.

### Obesity

If you are overweight and fit, Astanga is ideal for losing weight and toning the body. If you are overweight and unfit, Phil Beach, tutor at the British School of Naturopathy and Osteopathy, recommends you try other styles first. You can develop Astanga later to build fitness and stamina. Iyengar is valuable for its rigorous training, but all methods will gradually help to bring about weight balance by taking you to the root motivations of your drives.

### Reducing weight

Cecylia Hinds describes how yoga has helped her to reduce weight:
"When I started yoga in my late teens I was very overweight – almost 13 stone – and very unhappy. It transformed me. It was wonderful to be in a place where it felt non-competitive, yet you are challenging yourself. In classes everybody helps everybody else. My very first class was Iyengar, which was a lovely starting point from which to grow… I love Sivananda for the flow… Astanga for the speed and energy [but with] my body size, I couldn't have started with Astanga."

### Pregnancy

Yoga is excellent for pregnancy and postnatal wellbeing, but only in specialist, teacher-led classes. Ruth White, Iyengar teacher says: "Iyengar took me through three pregnancies with wisdom and care. Viniyoga would be excellent too."

Do not begin Astanga if you are pregnant, but if you are already practising, you may be able to introduce modifications with a teacher's guidance.

### Stress

All forms of yoga bring about restoration and balance. If you are exhausted, Viniyoga and Sivananda are ideal, and Astanga can be practised like T'ai Chi – as soft as a bird in flight. The mood of the practice can change. Viniyoga practice can be highly demanding and advanced, so there are no fixed rules. For people who need soothing and grounding, Sivananda is suitable because a session works from the head down, starting with a headstand and moving through to standing asanas at the end, the reverse of an Astanga Vinyasa sequence. If you are really wound up, like an unexploded bomb, Astanga Vinyasa is fantastic for pouring all of your energies into the practice to dissipate and surrender anxieties.

" If I wake up in a funny mood, yoga helps me transform it or sometimes even understand it. Especially with crying, it definitely moves something. " MAGGIE MOON

We are all individuals. If we engage in the appropriate practice and open ourselves up to yoga, we will feel different afterwards – always. All systems are healing and balancing and yoga schools will design courses for specific needs.

" We are not meant to be perfect. Nor are we meant to hold on to rigid positions. We are meant to flow in a universe that is constantly moving beneath our feet. "

JEAN HOUSTON

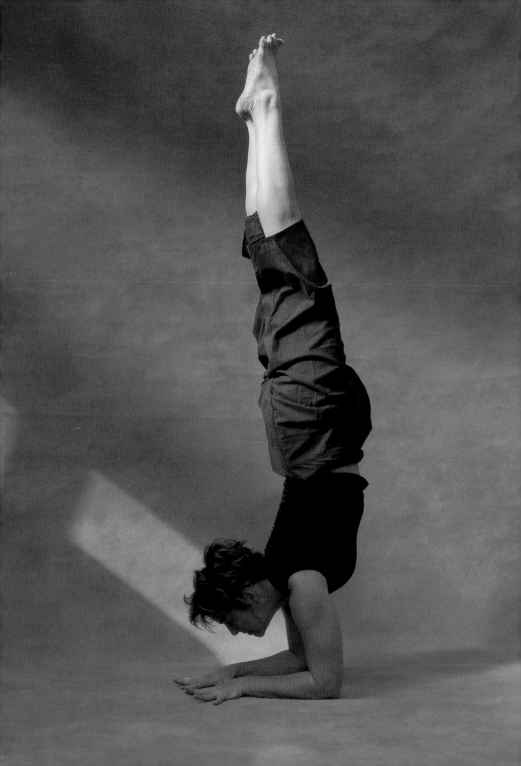

# The dance of the guna

"Guna" can be described as three qualities inherent in all material things. Observe an apple or some other fruit. In its unripe state it can be described as "rajasic". In its beautifully ripe state it can be described as "sattvic" – succulent, pure. In its overripe state, the apple is "tamasic". We can relate this to ourselves. When we want to dance or feel lively and mischievous, this active,

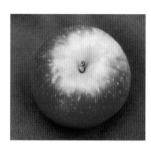

fiery state is rajasic; when we feel immobile, lethargic and heavy, we are tamasic; and when we achieve balance and clarity, we are in a sattvic state – just right, like Goldilocks and the porridge. In yoga we dance between the gunas, constantly exploring how to attain and maintain the sattvic state.

# Knowing your body type (dosha)

Our system should not have an excess or lack of anything in order to maintain harmony. Ayurveda, classical Indian medicine, expounds the concept of bodily doshas, consisting of air (vata), fire or bile (pitta) and phlegm or earth (kapha). It is the balance of these three qualities that maintains health. Because they are concerned with the relationship between mind and body, both Ayurveda and yoga – two facets of Tantra – assert that in order to be healthy, one must be happy and have mental clarity. Both systems emphasize preventative and maintenance medicine: participating in and taking responsibility for our health rather than relying on pills. The earliest sacred scripture in which Ayurveda is rooted is "artharva-veda", part of the Vedic heritage which records the principles of anatomy and medicine. The key is health from within as opposed to health from without.

We can be diagnosed as predominantly one dosha, or more usually two. Being aware of our body type can help us make good choices regarding diet, exercise and environment. What we take into our bodies can be nourishing, or a toxin if it does not absorb well. Coffee may stimulate a person who is predominantly kapha (earth ) in a beneficial way; it may set a predominantly vata (air) type spinning!

Below is a general outline of the doshas, but this is just a snapshot of a vast area of study, which also covers diet and other factors. Decide which dosha is dominant for you so you can follow the practice suggestions.

## Vata

*Characteristics:* light, thin build. Enthusiastic, excitable. Has bursts of energy, performing activities quickly. Quick to grasp new information. Tends to worry, changeable moods. Irregular hunger and digestion. Can be restless

*Element:* air. Vata controls movement in the body.

*Exercise:* needs to be soothing, grounding – Viniyoga or Sivananda, or other methods very softly approached. Needs steadiness, ample rest and lots of relaxation.

*Qualities of a balanced vata:* enthusiastic, happy, imaginative, alert.

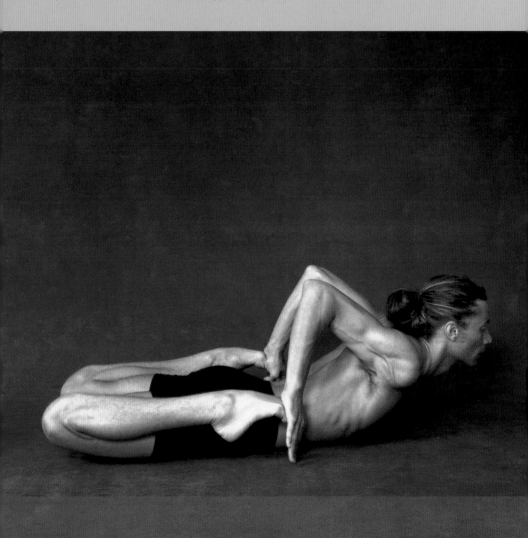

## Pitta

*Characteristics:* medium strength and endurance. Has sharp intellect and likes challenges. Articulate, bold, competitive, intense, tendency towards anger.
*Element:* fire. Pitta controls metabolism in the body. Strong digestion.
*Exercise:* sensitive constitution, so needs calming. Medium strength of practice. All yogas. Would love Astanga Vinyasa because of the challenge, but should practise it softly, with gentle breathing. Calming pranayama is valuable. Needs a balance between rest and activity. Viniyoga and Sivananda forms are suitable.
*Qualities of a balanced pitta:* warm, emotional, content, confident.

## Kapha

*Characteristics:* solid, powerful, physical. Steady energy, tranquil. Slow digestion, and tendency towards obesity and laziness. Affectionate, forgiving. Heavy sleep.
*Element:* earth. Kapha controls structure in the body.
*Exercise:* there is a need to "stoke the fire" so Astanga Vinyasa is ideal, and Iyengar. Needs regular, strong exercise.
*Qualities of a balanced kapha:* tranquil, relaxed, affectionate.

A Viniyoga session will adapt to suit all three doshas.

# Balance – the secret of health

Awareness of gunas and doshas brings more sensitivity to ourselves and to our environment, and can be helpful in monitoring how balanced we are – the secret of health. The yogic approach to health and fitness does not separate mind from body, but asks the question, "how can I be balanced, centred in all aspects of my being?" It is as important to soothe the emotions as it is to heal backache. One thing is certain: everything, including our bodies, is continually changing – we are not fixed and immutable "sculptures". For example, our skin completely renews itself every six weeks, and our skeleton every three months. (Despite this, scientists suggest that we use only about 3.5 per cent of our brainpower!)

To be balanced, we need qualities of all three doshas. Ayurvedic clinics recommend sun salutations followed by 15 minutes gentle yoga to harmonize the doshas. The practice should always include six ways of stretching: a forward bend, backbend, side stretch, twisting, a balancing posture (e.g. tree), an inversion (shoulderstand/headstand) with breathing awareness, equalizing inhalation and exhalation.

# Making the commitment

Despite the suggestions in this chapter, it is not so much a case of which method you choose as a question of how you practise – the quality of your attention and the ability to enter the moment. Swami Sivananda said, "An ounce of practice is worth tons of theory." When Swami Satyananda was asked the question, "What should I do if I don't have time to practise?" he replied, "If you don't have time to practise, why bother asking? One makes time to eat, sleep and work so why does it suddenly become difficult to make time for sadhana?"

Yoga is something you must experience. It is not to do with performance, or competition, but a means of self-enquiry. When we give time to yoga and meditation it gives us time back because it opens a door to eternity, beyond boundaries, like opening a window to a rush of butterflies.

The magical quality of committing oneself to a task with dedication is crystallized in the words of Goethe:

"Until one is committed there is hesitancy, the chance to draw back, always ineffectiveness. Concerning all acts of initiative (and creation), there is one elementary truth, the ignorance of which kills countless ideas and splendid plans: that the moment one definitely commits oneself, then Providence moves too... All sorts of things occur to help one that would never otherwise have occurred. The whole stream of events issues from the decision, raising in one's favour all manner of unforeseen incidents and meetings and material assistance, which no man could have dreamt would have come his way. Whatever you can do, or dream you can, begin it. Boldness has genius, power and magic in it. Begin it now."

# Preparing for practice

Always be comfortable and able to move freely in the clothes you are wearing. Wear natural fibres close to the skin. Astanga practitioners tend to expose as much skin as possible because toxins are eliminated through the skin when sweating. Iyengar practitioners also often expose the body in order to see clearly the direction and movement of bones and muscle groups. Sivananda and Viniyoga practitioners may wear loose, warmer clothing e.g. jogging bottoms and sweat tops. Always keep warm during practice.

Sunrise is the ideal time to practise before the business of the day and the cluttering of the mind sets in. Sun salutations greet the new day. A dynamic practice is good at the beginning of the day to energize and awaken, while a meditative practice is suited to the evenings to reflect upon the day and wind down.

The morning is also good because the stomach is empty (and it is easy to make excuses not to practise later in the day!). Leave a minimum of two hours after eating before practice.

The sun salutations should warm you up, but if you are very stiff modify them by bending the knees to soften the lower back in forward bends.

The room should be warm. Practise on a rubber yoga mat to get a good grip and avoid slipping. You may also like to have a blanket and an eye cushion to help relaxation at the end of a session.

It is good to bathe before and after practice out of respect for yourself (and your teacher!).

## Caution

Consult a doctor first if you have, or have had, any of the following: cancer, MS, epilepsy, high blood pressure, recent surgery, a neck or knee injury, ear or eye problems, HIV or AIDS.

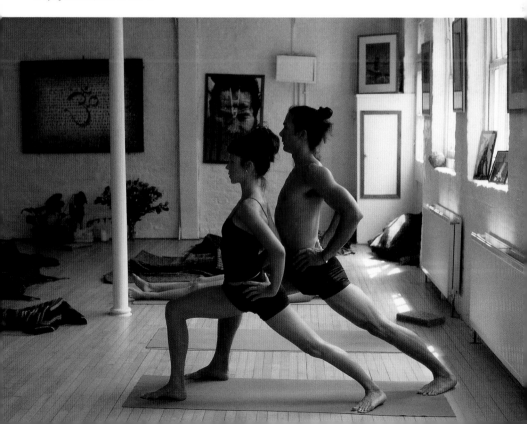

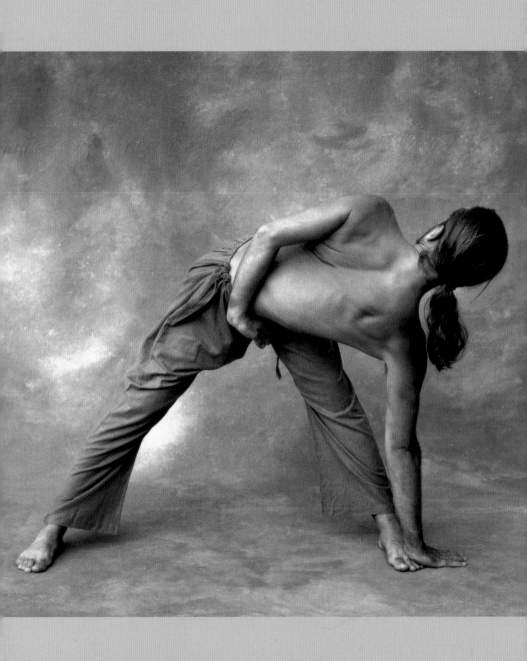

# VINIYOGA

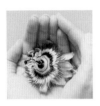

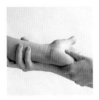

“ Yoga exists in the world because everything is linked... Yoga is relationship...The goal of yoga is peace, not power...peace cannot be attained through power, yet power is the result of peace. ” DESIKACHAR, *THE HEART OF YOGA*

Viniyoga is a complete yoga system based on the Yoga Sutra of Patanjali, which includes all Eight Limbs (see page 17). All Limbs are equally important, like each limb of an octopus: there is no emphasis placed on one aspect. Traditionally, yoga was practised one to one, not in large classes, with each individual given a specific programme tailored to their needs. Viniyoga works in this way. It is a personal, progressive approach, which has profoundly therapeutic powers. As suggested in the introduction, it can be helpful for specific needs, but also for those wanting a full range of practices including meditation.

# T. K. V. Desikachar

Desikachar, the son of Professor T. Krishnamacharya , was inspired directly by his father's teachings which he absorbed daily for 30 years starting in 1960 .

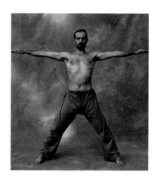

Originally a successful engineer, Desikachar stands with equal footing in East and West, representing the richness and depth of India with the advantages of a Western education. When asked by teacher Vanda Scaravelli what helped him most in his work, he replied "my engineering studies".

Stunned by the therapeutic effects of his father's teaching and much to his family's concern, Desikachar left his profession to become a yoga teacher, and to his surprise in the beginning, even the little he knew helped people. He began to teach in Europe in the1960s. Based in Chennai (formerly Madras), he continues to teach worldwide.

# Gill Lloyd, VINIYOGA BRITAIN

Gill Lloyd is the director of Viniyoga Britain and began practising yoga 28 years ago at the age of 28: "What yoga is really about is for people to feel good about themselves, and centred in themselves…Yoga does not take away the difficulties in life, but it can change our attitude and how we deal with the difficulties, so we don't get subsumed by them."

Gill has always been interested in religion. She studies yoga because she dislikes religious exclusivity and yoga allows a spiritual life without dogma. Viniyoga respects each individual and doesn't expect uniformity. Gill's teachers are T. K. V. Desikachar and Paul Harvey.

### Is Viniyoga suitable for everyone?

There is a myth that Viniyoga is a soft form of yoga, but it is also suitable for those who are fit and strong, and includes variations of headstand, handstand, elbowstand and advanced asanas. It is a refined form of yoga, suiting all abilities, whatever their needs. A practice can be as short as 15 minutes and as long as two hours, according to what is required and what is possible.

The only practice we do not follow is water cleansing techniques. We cleanse by air and fire depending on the individual's constitution [see doshas] – air with pranayama, fire with tapas (disciplined practice).

Jumping sequences are included in practice for children, who need lots of variety to keep them interested and enthusiastic.

**"** What is yoga after all? It is something we experience inside, **deep within our being**. Yoga is not an external experience. In yoga we try in every action to be as **attentive as possible** to everything we do. **"** DESIKACHAR

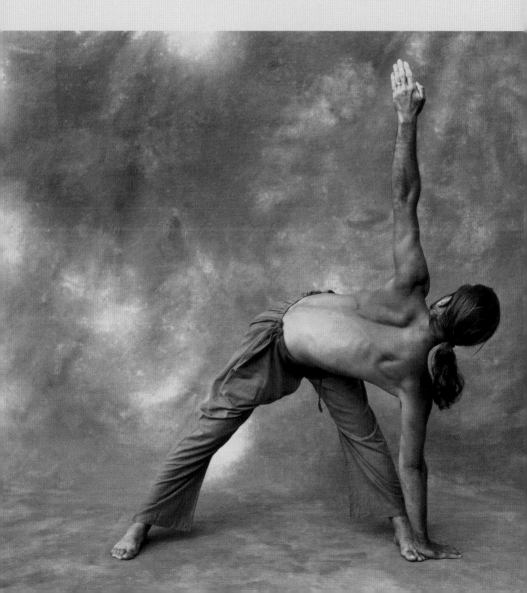

### Is it important to stay with one method?

If the method suits your needs, stay with it. Krishnamacharya said that if you are digging a well and you want to find water, you have to dig deeply in one spot and not dig many little holes everywhere.

### On gurus

Viniyoga does not have gurus, but "acharyas", hence the names Krishnamacharya and Desikachar(ya). Our real need is for good teachers, to mirror us and stop us kidding ourselves. Desikachar said an acharya is not someone who has a following, but one who can "show me the way", and he warned that following a guru can be another way of losing yourself!

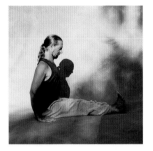

### On egos

Without the ego we would be a blob! The problem is when it gets out of balance, too inflated, egocentric, or too weak.

### Best way to learn

You need a good teacher, in a group or one to one. You will be given a programme to practise daily. You do what you can. Desikachar recommends a regular, daily practice, for it helps us to stay in the present moment. He recommends three things to help with the journey: first, tapas, heat or cleansing through asanas and pranayama; second svadhyaya, translating as self-study, asking the big questions who are we, and why are we here; third, suggested in the Yoga Sutra is the quality of Isvarapranidhana, which equates to acknowledging a higher force than ourselves.

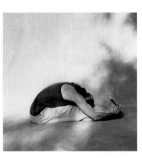

## The method

In Viniyoga, asana are tailored to suit all abilities. Pranayama (breathing practices) is always included; Vedic chanting can be part of the practice, and meditation when appropriate.

### Vinyasa krama

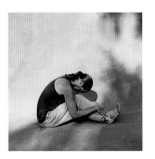

Vinyasa is defined as "to go towards a place"; "krama" is "step by step", implying a gradual, considered journey. Vinyasa krama is a step-by-step asana approach special to Viniyoga. The class structure reflects this, beginning with kneeling or standing, warming up with standing asanas developing into stronger postures, thus stretching the body safely. There is always a focus in each class, with an emphasis on building towards a particular posture, rather than a

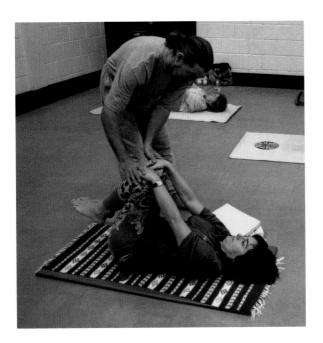

mixture of many postures. Like a symphony, the session sets a theme and develops it, building towards a crescendo, and then softening with quiet poses towards the end of the class. When necessary, rests are taken in Savasana (Corpse posture) at transitional points in the class. Final relaxation is short, since long relaxation is considered tamasic. The class concludes with seated breathing.

The practice flows and is never awkward. Much consideration is given to counterposes and modifications, to help people and to experience the psychological benefits.

### Pranayama

As Desikachar said, "Breathing means you care for yourself, you give some time to your own system to rejuvenate, and consciously you do it."

In Viniyoga, people are taught to work creatively with the breath, which is never lost sight of through the practice. A soft deep ujjayi (see page 24) is employed, each breath lasting longer than each movement. As in Astanga Vinyasa, breath is linked to asana, but it begins first, then the movement, with the breath continuing through the asana and beyond it, as if the posture is enveloped and contained inside the breath.

In Astanga Vinyasa breath and movement are the same length, but both systems concentrate the mind, monitoring the breath and its changes. Maintaining ujjayi has a soothing quality and draws the mind into the practice, linking asana (Third Limb) to pranayama (Fourth Limb). It is essential to breathe fully in all the poses; this keeps the practice safe and awareness engaged. Gill says that if you can't master the breath, you can't master the posture, and the breath is the first indicator of something going wrong. She adds, "If someone comes to me who is off the planet, they can gradually be led into a quieter space. A deeper exhale is calming, soothing; deeper inhalations stimulate and charge up the body." Teacher Andrew Payne suggests that if a person needs to be more assertive, breathing should be stronger, and if a person is too impulsive and needs to be calmer, a softer breath is encouraged. In Viniyoga, pranayama always completes the practice after a few minutes rest.

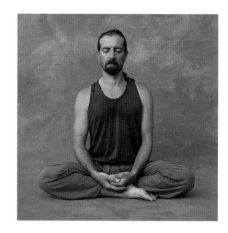

## Bandhas

When considerable breath control is mastered, and one is able to retain exhalation for a period of time, bandhas are sometimes, though not widely, taught. They are introduced in certain asanas, such as Downward Dog (see page 92) and are for skilful practitioners only. Classically, bandhas are taught with pranayama to direct energy.

## Suryanamaskara

One prepares for and builds up to the sun salutations in this method because they include some strong backbends and powerful leg movements. Similar to the Sivananda Suryanamaskara, the sequence is flowing and seamless, without the jumps present in the Astanga Vinyasa sequences.

## Meditation

In Viniyoga, meditation is taught on an individual basis, only when people want it. As Gill Lloyd explains, you don't "give it like a box of chocolates", but very gently, monitoring it step by step: "...you have to be really respectful of the person you are teaching... Watching the breath in class is a meditation. It is happening in class. If you are involved in class, it is a meditation. Meditation is not separate, it is the degree of focus and involvement in what you are doing."

**"** ... the quality of breath is the clearest indication
of the quality of our asana practice. **"**

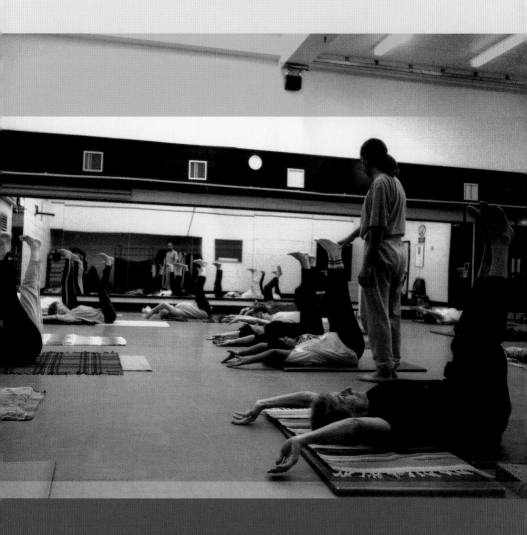

# Practice

The following practice is a sample Viniyoga practice which flows in a step-by-step progression to balance the whole body and mind. Rest between asanas so that your breathing returns to normal. The ujjayi breath is described on page 24.

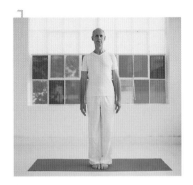

**1.** Stand quietly focused in samasthiti (standing steadily), the first classical standing asana. Take a soft, long ujjayi breath.

**2.** Inhale and raise your arms up over your head.

**3.** Exhale and fold into a forward bend.

Repeat the cycle eight times.

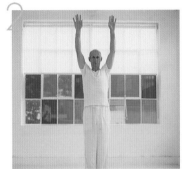

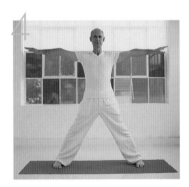

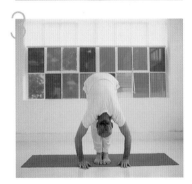

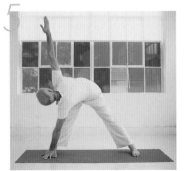

**4.** Step the legs 3 feet apart and stretch the arms to each side. Inhale and lengthen through your arms.

**5.** Exhale and, bending from the hips, move your left hand to your right foot. Repeat cycle 12 times, moving to alternate sides.

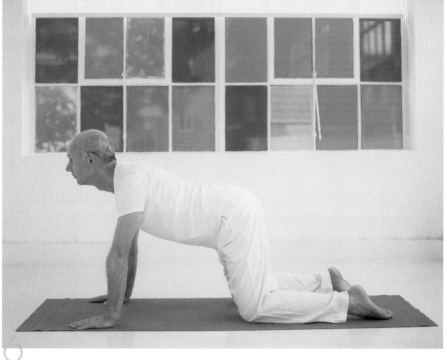

**6.** Come into a tabletop position, i.e. kneel with knees beneath your hips and hands beneath your shoulders, lifting your tailbone upwards. This is the Cat pose. Inhale, arch the spine and look up.

**7.** Exhale, raise the hips back into the Downward Dog stretch (see page 92). Repeat cycle six times, fluidly moving from Cat to Dog.

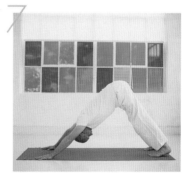

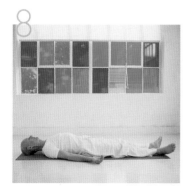

**8.** Savasana, Corpse pose. Relax in Savasana, the resting pose, observing your breathing until it returns to normal.

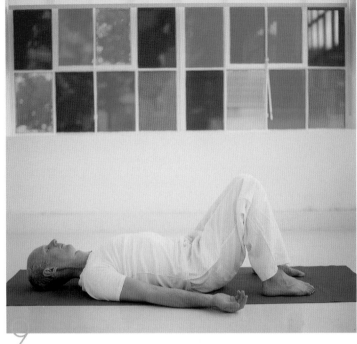

**9.** Two foot support: "dwi pada peetham". Lie semi-supine with your knees raised and your feet hip-width apart and parallel. Relax your arms by your sides, soften the back of the neck and broaden across your shoulders.

**10.** Inhale and raise your hips. Exhale and lower your hips to the floor. Repeat cycle six times.

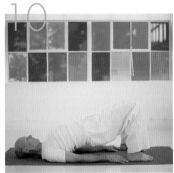

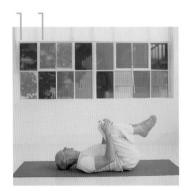

**11.** Knees to chest: "mut apanasana". On release, hug your legs into your abdomen, resting and breathing a soft, ujjayi breath.

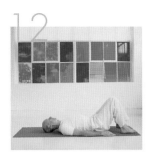

**12.** Lie supine with your knees raised and your feet hip-width apart and parallel. Relax your arms by your sides, soften the back of the neck and broaden across your shoulders.

**13.** Inhale and raise your arms over your head.

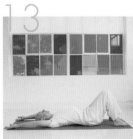

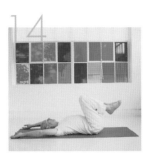

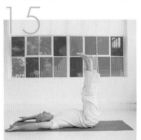

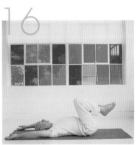

**14.** Exhale and lift your feet off the floor, tucking your thighs into your abdomen.

**15.** Inhale and stretch your legs up towards the sky, straightening them.

**16.** Exhale and bend your knees, tucking your thighs into your abdomen.

**17.** Inhale and place your feet on the floor, returning to the semi-supine position.

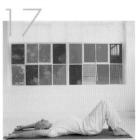

**18.** Exhale and lower your arms down to your sides.

Repeat cycle four times.

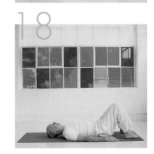

**19.** From the supine position, raise straightened legs up to the sky, open your arms wide. (Abdominal awareness is recommended here for core support to protect the lower back.) Inhale deeply.

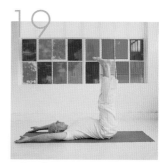

**20.** Exhale, lower straightened legs to the right, if possible placing your toes in your right hand. Turn your head and gaze to the left. Take 12 breaths. Inhale, raise the legs back up with feet pointing to the sky. Repeat on the left side, one cycle only.

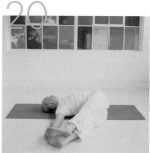

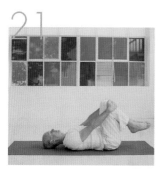

**21.** Knees to chest: mut apanasana. Resting limber. On release, hug your legs into your abdomen, resting and breathing a soft, ujjayi breath.

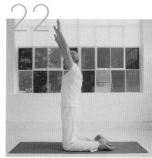

**22.** Come into a raised kneeling position placing the knees hip-width apart. Inhale and lift your arms up in front of you.

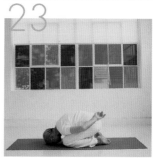

**23.** Exhale and fold your body forward into a child's pose, i.e. curl up, place your brow on the floor and bring your arms down behind your back.

Repeat cycle (22 and 23) six times with fluid movement and deep, soft ujjayi breathing.

You may choose to end this practice with nadishodana (see opposite). If not, your practice is now complete. Take a short rest in Savasana Corpse posture.

# Nadishodana – Alternate Nostril Breathing

Rest before beginning this pranayama practice. You must learn this with a teacher. Sit as upright as possible. Breathe freely. Make the mrgi mudra gesture by curling in the index and middle finger of the right hand so the thumb and fourth finger can be used on either side of the nose to close the nostrils.

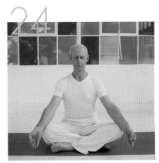

**1.** Inhale through both nostrils.

**2.** Close the right nostril at the sinus bridge with the right thumb, exhale through the left nostril. Count to four.

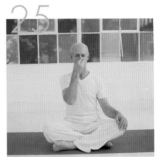

**3.** Inhale through the left nostril while counting to four.

**4.** Close left nostril with the fourth finger of right hand, exhale through the right nostril, counting to four. Inhale through the right nostril counting to four.

**5.** Close the right nostril, exhale through the left nostril counting to four. Inhale through the left nostril counting to four.

**6.** Release the right nostril and exhale completely.

Your practise is now complete. Sit and allow the body/mind to settle.

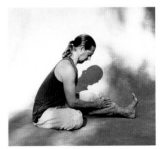

# Maha mudra – the Great Seal

The Great Seal is a life-enhancing classical mudra (gesture), which works with energy, harnessing the three bandhas and linking up a fourth, jiva, whereby the tongue tip is placed at the junction between the hard and soft palate, sealing energy in the body.

**1.** Stretch out your right leg, bend your left knee and press your anus with the left heel. Catch your right foot with both hands.

**2.** Inhale, retain the breath (kumbhaka) and hold for as long as is comfortable. Then change sides.

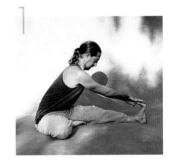

**Modification** (right): slightly bend the outstretched leg if necessary to avoid straining the back.

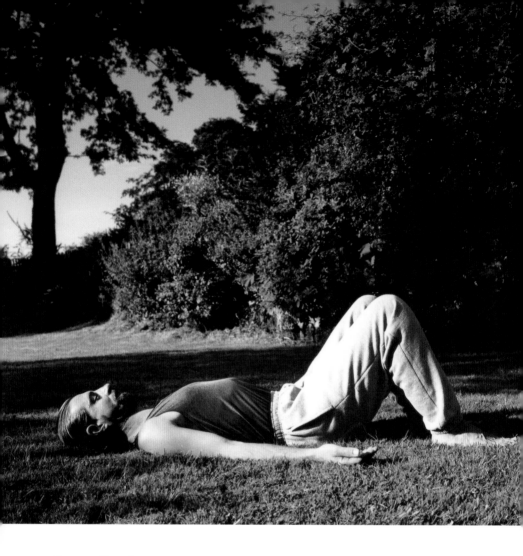

# Case Study

ANDREW PAYNE teaches Viniyoga and runs a gardening business. He began practising yoga about 15 years ago when he was 24, prompted by his wife, to ease discomfort from a back injury. He has specialized in Viniyoga for nine years.

Brought up by his mother and grandmother, Andrew has had strong feminine influences in his life. He recognizes that when young he was full of innate arrogance and pride, which may have been protective bravado. He grew up in an underprivileged environment and as a child he questioned everything. By his mid-teens he used drugs and alcohol to mask the questioning, but as it didn't go away he eventually decided to do something about it, and found that the journey which started with back pain led to the heart.

He emphasizes that Viniyoga is not a soft form of yoga: "The things I'm facing up to are inside my body, psychologically, emotionally, intellectually, such as, 'is my heart closed?' If you are open, Viniyoga embraces everything: heart, mind and soul. Yoga is like a torch that shines inside, and led by a teacher we need to go into the dark places.

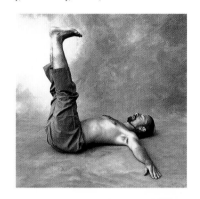

As a teacher you continue to have individual sessions with your teacher, to ripen spiritually. Yoga brings freedom, not from life, but freedom within life. It enriches and embraces life rather than denies it."

Andrew enjoys his gardening business which is solitary, "earthed" and linked to nature. Two years ago, while working up a tree, he fell out and landed on an iron gatepost. Rushed by paramedics to hospital and thought to have a punctured lung, he found the psychological impact of nearly dying was huge, but is convinced that yoga got him back to work within four weeks: "Commonplace miracles are happening every day. You plant an acorn – it grows into a huge oak tree!"

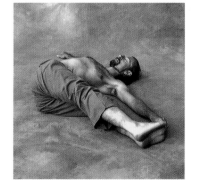

It is Andrew's belief that there has never been, for the greater mass of humanity, such an opportunity to change if we want to, and he hopes that the leisure time which many now have can be used spiritually for self-improvement. He stresses the yoga view of dividing our time between four qualities for a balanced life: "utta", our needs; "kama", sweetness, pleasures; "dharma", our duties; and "moksha", liberation.

Andy teaches people between the ages of 17 and 77, from students to people in hospices: "Viniyoga respects the individual's needs, where they are and what they are capable of, and where they can go."

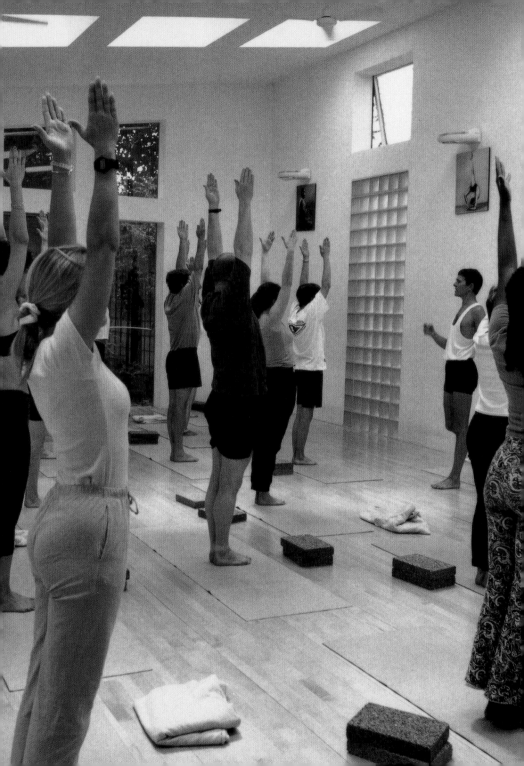

# IYENGAR

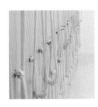

**"**...bring the **mind** to rest on each and every cell...each cell has to appear to me as if it has an intellectual eye.**"** IYENGAR

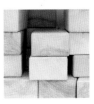

IYENGAR YOGA SPEAKS DIRECTLY TO THE BODY in a wonderful language that opens the channels between intellect and feeling, synthesizing all aspects of the human being. Through attention to the body, the mind is brought closer to the self. A precise and rigorous approach, Iyengar yoga's aim is the refinement of inner intelligence through physical and mental training. Through meditation you can reach a deep state of awareness as though you can feel every single part of your body. Constantly exploring the technology of the body and the mysteries of the mind, the originator of this approach to yoga, Iyengar, has sought relentlessly to "make every cell shine with vibrant energy, and to make them all say unanimously and with one voice a resounding 'yes!' to life and light".

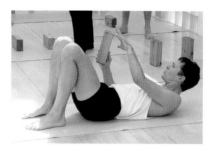

# Illness

You can practise Iyengar yoga while suffering from an illness, as long as the appropriate class is chosen. If feverish, however, you should rest. Iyengar yoga schools organize special classes for those who are ill or injured and if you feel unwell during a class there is always something helpful you can do. For instance, if you suffer from fatigue, you can sit kneeling until it passes; and if you feel nauseous, you can go into a standing forward bend, folding the elbows.

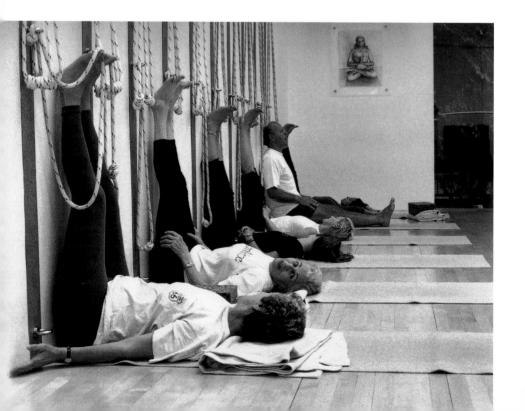

# Iyengar

B.K.S. Iyengar, an "architect of the body", was born in 1918, in Bellur, near Bangalore. He was the eleventh child of a poor Brahmin family. Unlike Desikachar, the founder of Viniyoga, he was not born into a family of yogis. His father, a schoolmaster, with whom he felt a mystical connection, died when he was nine and much of Iyengar's early life was hard, with periods of illness and isolation.

In 1934, suffering from tuberculosis, Iyengar joined Krishnamacharya's yoga school in Mysore, southern India in order to regain his health. Here he received strict training in asanas and pranayama, although at first he could not even touch his knees with his fingers. This marked the turning point of Iyengar's life.

In 1936, Krishnamacharya travelled round the northern districts of Mysore with his students, and a doctor, noticing Iyengar's unlimited enthusiasm, invited him to teach in Poona, Maharashtra. So in 1937 Iyengar arrived in Poona as a yoga teacher with about four rupees, two shirts, some dhotis (loincloths) and a bedroll.

Faced with the challenge of teaching, and believing knowledge is gained through experience, he practised up to 12 hours a day, continuing his thorough and rigorous approach to yoga. After many years of teaching he began to read yoga texts.

When asked at what point yoga becomes joyful, Iyengar replies: "When one practises with effortless effort."

" All these yogic postures bring intelligence to flow in the system like a river as a single unit. Then the mind, the self, the body, they all unite together... To awaken the intelligence of the body, one must keep the essence and foundation principles, then explore using the 'human feeling' approach... In this technological world we have lost the resonance of the spine. " IYENGAR

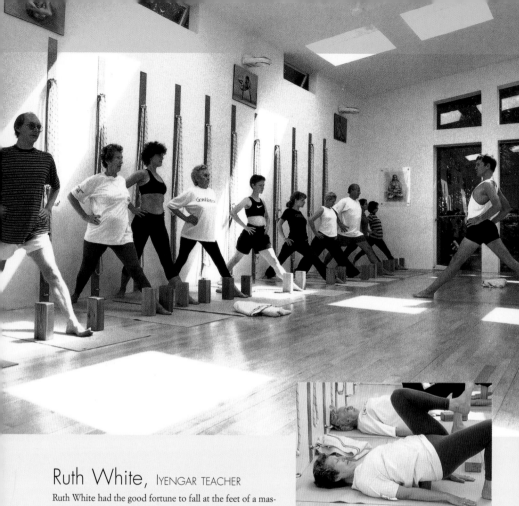

# Ruth White, IYENGAR TEACHER

Ruth White had the good fortune to fall at the feet of a master – Iyengar – in her late teens when suffering from chronic back problems. Iyengar alleviated her pain and showed Ruth ways to strengthen her back. Over the years he has taken her through three pregnancies with wisdom and care. She practises yoga because it lifts her spirits and brings wellbeing. For her, the meaning of yoga is peace and harmony.

*Is Iyengar yoga suitable for everyone?*
Yes, under an experienced and caring teacher who will adapt the postures to suit the individual's needs.

*Is it important to stay with one method?*

Yoga is about unity and is taught by many people. It is up to the practitioner to find the right practice. I was taught personally by Iyengar and am greatly inspired by his teaching, but I have to teach from the heart and need to adapt to the ever-changing needs of students.

*On gurus*

They help you to fly, but using your own wings.

*On egos*

Ignore the ego and attend to this moment, especially if you are a teacher.

*Best way to learn*

Find a teacher with whom you communicate well, so that the knowledge flows between you. Everyone needs to practise.

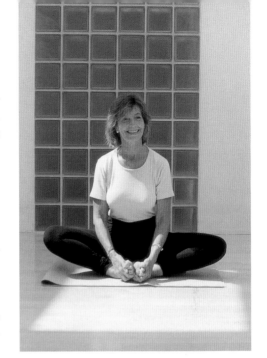

# The method

Iyengar yoga involves precise alignments and postures, and makes use of props and modifications. Suitable for middle-aged people, it can also be tailored to suit particular needs and abilities: "There is absolutely no age limit to sex or yoga... the self has no age. The mind introduces fear: it is the mind which has to be cultivated." Iyengar, London masterclass, 1985

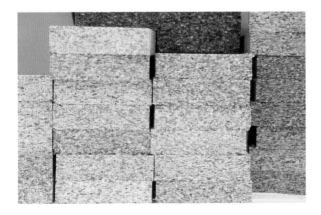

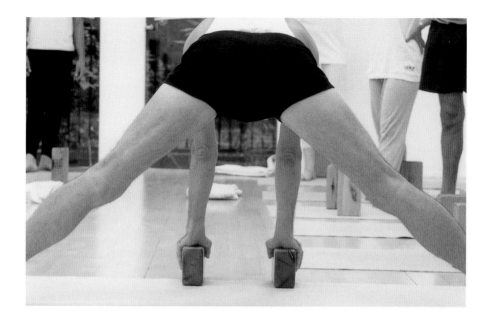

## Pranayama

Most of us don't breathe properly. We need to breathe more deeply, opening the ribcage. Breathing freely increases our awareness naturally. It is important not to intellectualize about the breath, but rather to feel the process of breathing. In class, Iyengar tells students to breathe normally. Synchronized breathing with postures begins straightaway, and breathing is through the nose. Iyengar is well known for saying, "The mouth is for eating, the nose is for breathing. If you breathe through your mouth I will feed you through your nose!"

Advanced pranayama is taught to practitioners with two to three years' experience, and to people with special needs. Because it is an advanced practice it should be approached with caution.

## Bandhas

In Iyengar yoga, bandhas are not at first taught with asanas, but are built gradually into the structure and architecture of the dynamic posture alignment. The mula bandha, the more energetic bandha technique, can be included (see page 25).

The bandhas are also important in pranayama practice, particularly jalandhara , the restraint of the throat (see page 24).

### Suryanamaskars

In the early days Iyengar himself practised sun salutations. Now, although they are a feature of Iyengar yoga, Tadasana, the Mountain pose, is used between postures.

" As you are inhaling, feel that you are drawing the Lord in the form of breath into your lungs so that you are one with the Lord who is known as the universal spirit. Then when you are holding the breath, you and the Lord are wedded together, divinely united and as long as that feeling is there, hold on. " IYENGAR, LONDON MASTERCLASS, 1985

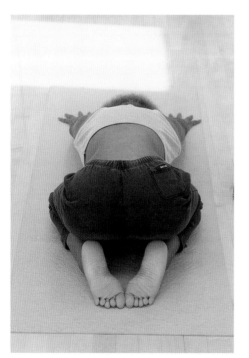

### Meditation

In Iyengar's words: "We have to master the known [body] fully in order to master the unknown [soul]". Yoga is dynamic meditation and Iyengar describes the poses as his prayers. In yoga the body is trained rigorously to surrender the ego. Meditation should bring a sense of fullness, and "all-one-ness", not depletion or separation. All the postures lead to the opening up of an inner world in a process of pratyahara – sense-withdrawal (the Fifth Limb). Iyengar says that we have been given the body in order to realize the temple of the self. If practitioners concentrate sufficiently in meditation, the mind becomes "a sea without waves".

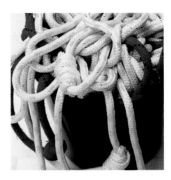

## Practice

A typical Iyengar class starts with students' questions, which are answered through the yoga practice. Although a specific class structure can be helpful, a teacher responding to a need cannot keep to one format because the need is ever changing. For example, backbends release negativity and bring energy; forward bends are more soothing. The following practice session is based on Ruth White's class for people who are tired after work. This demonstration therefore begins with a number of backbends, recuperative postures that can be developed further in a longer class. Throughout your practice, breathe with awareness. Be wholehearted. There must be complete attention to what you are doing.

**Bob Waters** is an Iyengar teacher. He started at 22 after returning from India unwell. To help him to regain health, his mother took him to a yoga class, and he has been practising ever since. He says of Iyengar, "It's not eastern gymnastics."

“ Reduced to our own body, our first instrument,
we learn to play it,
drawing from it maximum resonance and harmony. ”

SIR YEHUDI MENUHIN, TAUGHT BY IYENGAR

# " The intelligence

is brought to observe **moment** to moment. "

IYENGAR, LONDON MASTERCLASS, 1985

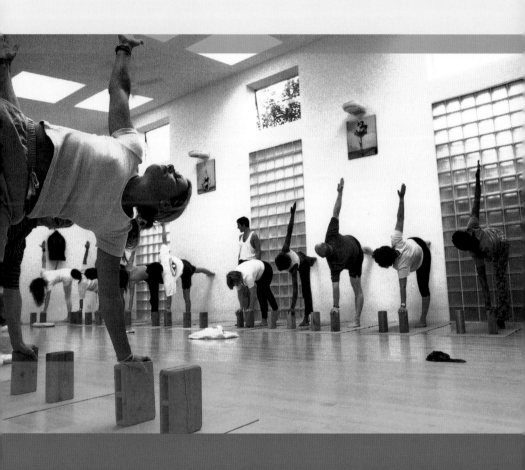

# Dome

**1.** The back is arched over a dome shape. The teacher checks the position of the neck and, if necessary, places a block behind the back of the neck to avoid tension there.

**2.** The collarbones are widened out, shoulder blades are drawn together, and the shoulders softened. Blocks beneath the ankles and buttocks diminish the arch in the back.

**3.** Remain in that position for several minutes. Then remove the props and lie semi-supine.

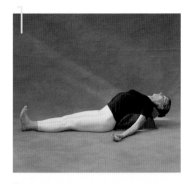

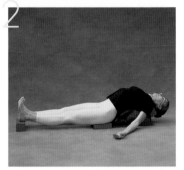

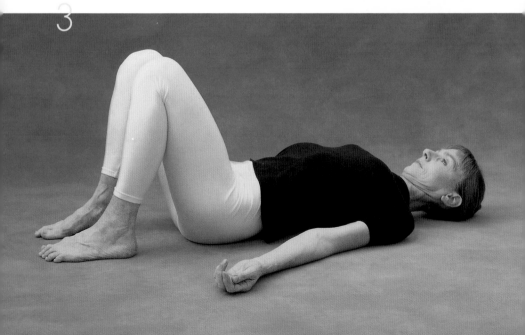

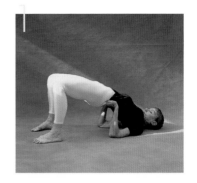

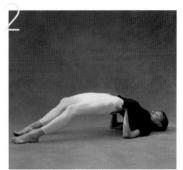

## Sethubandasana – BRIDGE POSTURE

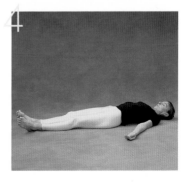

To prepare for the Bridge posture, bend your knees and, avoiding strain in your neck, press your upper arms into the floor.

**1.** Raise your tailbone. Push your inner heels into the floor and raise your pelvis, stretching up the skin on the sides of your ribs.

**2.** Now straighten your legs. The top of your chest moves towards your chin, your collarbones move towards your ears. Shoulders and back of the neck rest on the floor. Roll the outside of your upper arms into the floor.

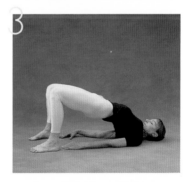

**3.** Keep your legs bent if there is too much pressure on the lower spine.

**4.** Exhaling, come down and stretch out your legs. Then draw the abdominal area in and up, lengthening yourself from the ribcage to the pelvic girdle.

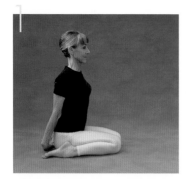

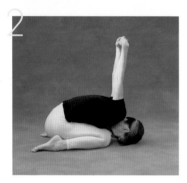

## Supta Vajrasana – RECUPERATION POSE

This posture opens up two areas: the groin and the top of the chest, so energy levels rise and the inner organs work more efficiently.

**1.** Sit between your feet. Interlock your fingers behind your back, raising your collarbones higher and higher. The tops of your feet should touch the floor. Do not let your feet turn out sideways.

**2.** With hands clasped behind your back, fold into a forward bend, raising your arms up behind you. Breathe normally.

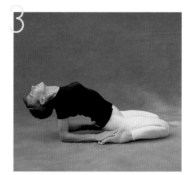

**3.** Inhaling, come up to a kneeling position, and arch your back on to your elbows. Do not tremble. Stretch away from the groin.

**4.** If this is difficult, lie all the way down instead.

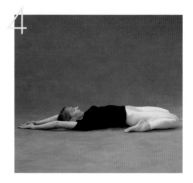

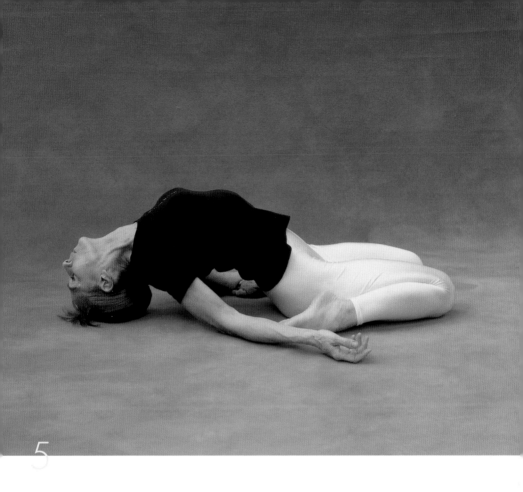

**5.** For advanced practitioners only, lift the top of your chest upwards and place the top of your head on the floor. Expand the heart, throat and lung area.

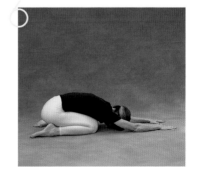

**6.** Rest in child's pose, curling the upper body over the thighs.

When you have done this, notice if your energy levels have changed, and observe the dominant guna (see page 37). Soon you will begin to notice the effects of asanas, and begin to know when to practise each one. Now you should practise standing asanas.

## Tadasana – MOUNTAIN POSTURE

Observe yourself in Tadasana, even if you have been practising for years. Become aware of your feet, extend your heels backwards from the inner arch, adjust your big toe from the centre, taking weight into every toe. Spread wide the balls of your feet. Balance the weight equally through all four corners of your feet. Activate the muscles in your legs and raise the kneecaps. Breathe normally. Lift up from the pelvic floor, continually. The spine ascends, the legs descend. Lift the base of your skull. Broaden your collarbones and lift your whole ribcage upwards.

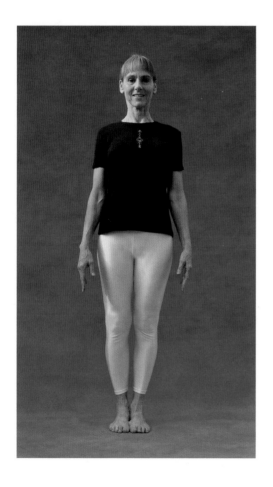

" When you're turning the **body** you should also turn the mind. Stretch both sides of the body, like wings. Stretch your skin from the inner ankles up to the hips. Adjust yourself **connectively** to the skin. "

IYENGAR, LONDON MASTERCLASS, 1985

# Trikonasana – TRIANGLE POSTURE

For the Triangle posture, start from Tadasana. Inhale, exhale, jump your feet 3 feet apart, straighten your legs, lengthen your spine, and broaden across your chest. Extend your arms.

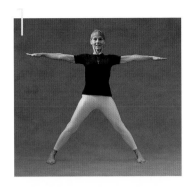

**1.** Turn your right foot inwards 15 degrees, and the ball of your left foot out 90 degrees. Draw your right hip back, and open out your right shoulder. There is a strong action going on: you are pulling back the whole of the right side of your body.

**2.** Exhaling, stretch out your right side as much as you can, lengthening the right of your waist, pressing your left buttock forwards and rotating your thigh muscles outwards. Ground the balls of your feet, press your inner and outer heels into the mat. Do not wrinkle your left waist.

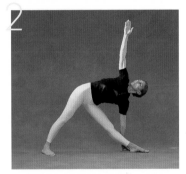

**3.** Catch your left ankle with your left hand or place your finger-tips on the floor. The entire plate of your right foot should be on the floor. Gaze up to your left thumb.

**4.** If this posture is too intense, place a block beside your left foot and rest the left hand on it.

**5.** Inhale and come up without trembling, getting feedback from your body all the time. Now repeat the posture on the right side.

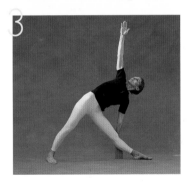

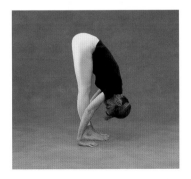

Rest between postures in a standing forward bend, to restore and soothe the brain. Breathe normally. Inhale, come up, exhale, jump back to Tadasana.

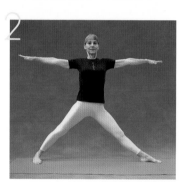

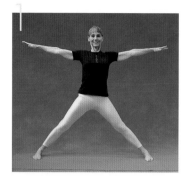

# Utthita Parsvakonasana
– EXTENDED ANGLE POSE

**1.** Breathe in and jump your feet 4 feet apart. Extend your arms wide like wings.

**2.** Turn your right foot inwards, turn your left foot outwards 90 degrees. Exhaling, without losing the grip of your right foot, bend the left knee. Push down through your right heel.

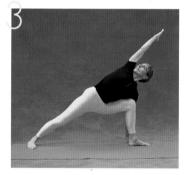

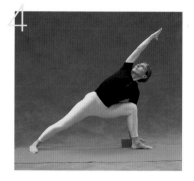

**3.** Exhaling, take the fingertips of your left hand to the floor, outside your left foot. Then, in this tremendously strong movement, take your right arm over your head – your knee is directly above your ankle, shinbone vertical. Press strongly into your right foot and straighten the right leg. Look up. Breathe normally.

**4.** If the posture is too intense, use a block for the left hand. Aim to create a diagonal line through the right side of your body.

Breathe in and come up. Now repeat on the right side. Return to Tadasana. Make sure your knees are pointing forwards. Extend your heels backwards from the inner arch. Lengthen the leg muscles, making the legs strong and firm.

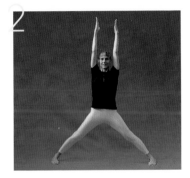

# Virabhadrasana – WARRIOR POSE

**1.** Take a deep inhalation and jump your feet 4 feet apart, arms wide open with the palms facing upwards to roll back the shoulders.

**2.** Raise your arms up over your head, turn the left heel in, revolving the left hip towards the right side of your groin. Spin your right hip back, lengthening the right side of your waist.

**3.** As you exhale, bend your right leg. Breathe normally, sharing equal weight between both legs.

Inhale and return to centre, keeping your arms raised. Now repeat on the left side. Inhale, straighten both legs and return to Tadasana.

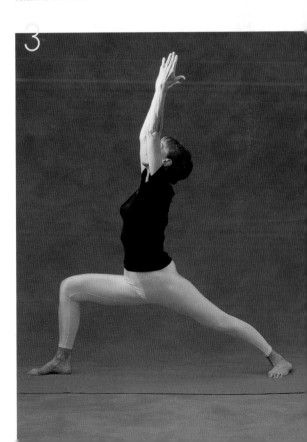

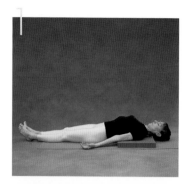

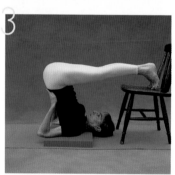

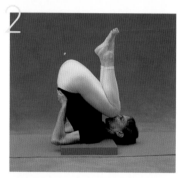

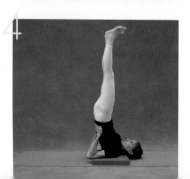

## Sarvangasana – SHOULDERSTAND

**1.** Create a firm, padded base for your shoulders and your upper back, allowing the head to lie lower than the shoulders.

**2.** Press your hands on your hips firmly. Inhale and raise your legs, curling them into your body and supporting your back firmly with your hands.

**3.** Stretch your legs as straight as you can, pressing them together. Still supporting your back, exhale, dropping your legs over on to a chair or bench for a supported Halasana posture. Remain in this position for two minutes if comfortable. Breathe normally. This is a strongly calming posture: "ploughing the soil of the mind to dig out conditioned thoughts."

**4.** Now raise the legs up, keeping the back and the legs as straight as you can. Lift the balls of the feet to the ceiling. Remain in this position for a full minute if comfortable (time spent in an asana can be extended with the help of a teacher).

## Relaxation

**1.** Matsyasana – Fish pose. Outstretch the legs, or butterfly open the hips pressing the soles of the feet together. Arch the spine, resting the top of your head on the floor. Breathe normally, expanding the chest area.

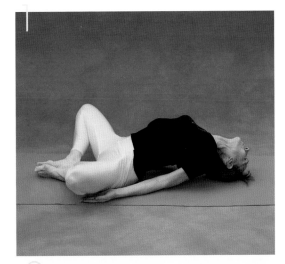

**2.** Savasana – Corpse posture. Roll softly down into Corpse posture to prepare for final relaxation. Make sure you are warm and comfortable. With your body at ease now and muscles soft, let all sounds go into a haze. Rest in your quiet centre.

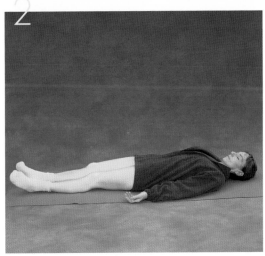

“All these postures **lead to the invisible**,

take one to the extreme peace which we call truth.”

IYENGAR, 1976

# Case Studies

JEAN HALL, a dancer and yoga teacher, came to yoga at the age of 12. As she watched her mother practise she was intrigued by the concept of positive energy breathed into the body, and the power of the mind:

"I practise the Astanga series with different influences using my Iyengar training. It's important to explore, to be open. We have many different qualities within ourselves and the practice is a way of integrating these different qualities. How we practise is what is important, to bring about balance."

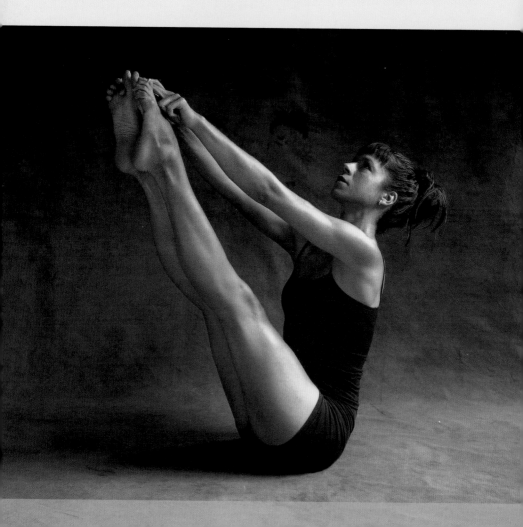

**ANN ALLEN**, who started yoga to cure her varicose veins after having children, practises Iyengar for depth of alignment and Astanga for fun:

"Combining the two is superb: the precision of Iyengar and the flow of breath and fluidity of Astanga... but we must be sure to learn alignment deeply too."

**ANNE PALMER**, head of Newcastle Shiatsu School, England, recommends Iyengar for a wide variety of people: those who don't like aerobic exercise, those who may be injured or in recovery, and those who like precision and calmness, but who seek a strong practice.

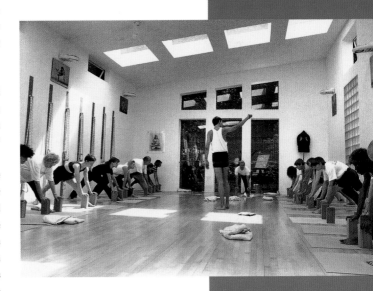

**AMRITA** is an ordained Buddhist who uses yoga as a way of deepening his Buddhist practice. He has 15 years' experience of Iyengar yoga:

"It is important to practise asana with awareness. Iyengar yoga develops precision and alignment, which means we can open the body safely. As the poet John Keats said, 'truth is beauty, beauty is truth'. It is our duty to express the truth as beautifully as possible. We should strive to make each asana as beautiful as possible both externally and internally, so although we may do Trikonasana ten thousand times, if we aim to make the pose as beautiful as possible we align ourselves with truth.

Most of the time we dissipate our valuable life energy through our eyes, mouth and through our ungainly movements. By placing attention on the bandhas, breath and drishtis we seal our energy within which gives us greater freedom to redirect our life energy towards awakening our potential. Awareness of the body leads to more beautiful movement."

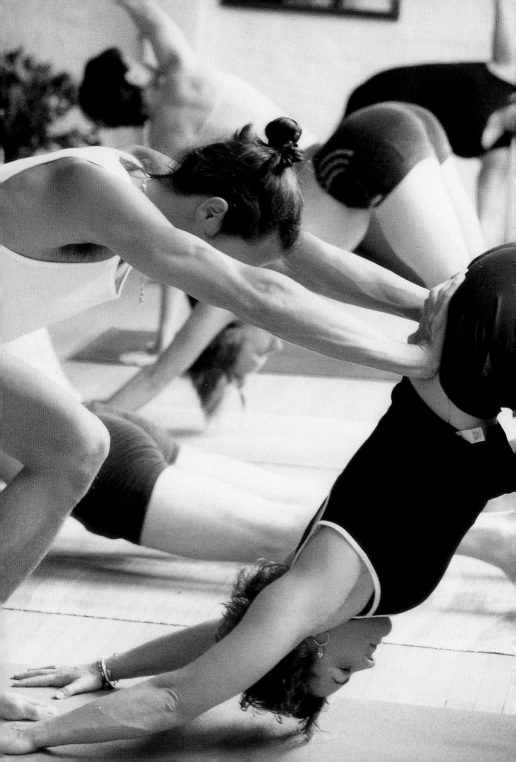

# ASTANGA VINYASA

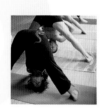

“ A fluid sequence of **asanas**, threaded together like a garland of flowers on to the unbroken thread of breath. ”

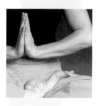

Astanga Vinyasa yoga takes its name from "ast" meaning eight, "anga" meaning limbs and "vinyasa" meaning breath-synchronized movement. It is a dynamic, physical form of yoga, deciphered from ancient Sanskrit by Krishnamacharya. It's fantastic for young people and those with lots of energy. Gingi Lee, yoga teacher, was brought up with martial arts. He became a black-belt karate practitioner, trained by his father, a "sensei" (master). Gingi, now devoted to Astanga Vinyasa yoga, says, "In karate you learn how to fight outwardly. In yoga the battles you fight are within yourself."

Astanga Vinyasa focuses and directs your energy as if you are stoking up a fire to purify the body. It greatly improves shape and tone and can be described as deep meditation in movement.

You have to practise Astanga Vinyasa to discover its depth and richness, for yoga is experiential. David Swenson, a practitioner of more than 25 years, is convinced of its benefits: "When I don't practise, I notice my life is much more difficult... It's the place in my mind where I go when I'm practising that keeps me practising – I am not the body... Ultimately it's an internal practice."

# Sri K. Pattabhi Jois

Born in 1915, Sri K. Pattabhi Jois grew up in a modest household near Mysore. One of nine children, his father was a landowner and astrologer. At the early age of 12 he began studies with Professor T. Krishnamacharya with whom he remained for 18 years until 1945.

Pattabhi Jois studied Sanskrit and Vedanta philosophy at Mysore Maharaja Sanskrit College, where he became head of the yoga department. He became most famous for Astanga Vinyasa yoga, which is said to have originated from an ancient Sanskrit text, the *Yoga Korunta*, written by Rishi Vamana. Pattabhi Jois worked closely with Professor Krishnamacharya to decipher and collate the yoga "series" and in 1958 he published the *Yoga Mala*. "Malas" are fresh jasmine garlands strung together daily by women in India: the aim in Astanga yoga is to develop a fluid sequence of asanas, threaded on to the breath. The book describes the primary foundation series of Astanga Vinyasa yoga, which has three series altogether. The primary series is known as Yoga Chikitsa (yoga therapy) and is designed to realign, detoxify and strengthen the system.

In 1948 Pattabhi Jois taught local Brahmin boys, and later, in the 1960s, he began to teach Europeans, dedicating himself to teaching Astanga Vinyasa.

# Liz Lark, ASTANGA VINYASA TEACHER

At school an innovative PE teacher gave us some introductory yoga sessions and the feeling of mental involvement in the body immediately struck me, relating to psychological wellbeing in sport. As an international basketball player, I was interested in mental focus, which yoga develops, as a means of harnessing and directing potential. I approached yoga with a love of physicality and creative movement combined with a spiritual enquiry for a path without dogma or institutionalisation. Yoga anchors me and liberates me and in London or any big city, this is essential.

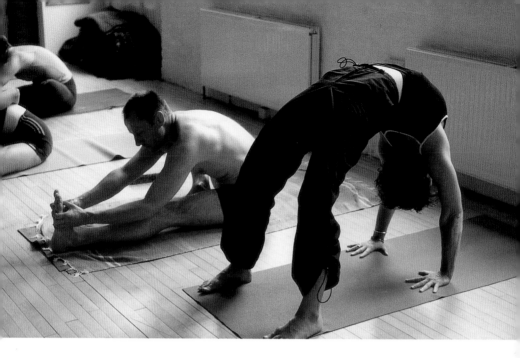

### Astanga Vinyasa for everyone

We are always changing. Practice can be adapted to suit individual needs –
that is what Krishnamacharya taught. Yoga grows organically through our life.

### Staying with one method

To explore, to climb inside the practice and grow in it, you need to commit to
one method, otherwise there is no anchor. Within that framework, like swimming in the sea, visit other islands and glean from them, but go empty-hand-
ed. Integrate the knowledge back into your practice. Iyengar alignment feeds
Astanga practice. Sivananda's softness and open-heartedness is valuable and
increases our concern with the world. Viniyoga's way of adapting the methods allows us always to practise something, even with injury, and Viniyoga's
breath monitoring and awareness is masterful.

Following a clearly defined method gives us a structure to explore freedom within a form.

### On gurus

The guru of many practitioners is Sri K. Pattabhi Jois. It is valuable to go to
the source, the master, but one could say that, if we are open, everyone we
meet can be a guru, a "bringer of light". Ultimately, we must enquire within.

*On egos*

Biba Logan said, "I confront the ego every time I step on my mat." Astanga Vinyasa is a warrior yoga. It empowers you and builds a healthy ego. From this basis we move beyond the boundaries of the ego, or conscious personality, towards the self, or soul, described in Jungian terms as "a place of solid ground within". It is unhealthy to try to stamp out the ego. In Astanga Vinyasa, as in all the yogas, we must be brave, because we are playing with fire – our energies, our potential, our shadows – channelling and sublimating them.

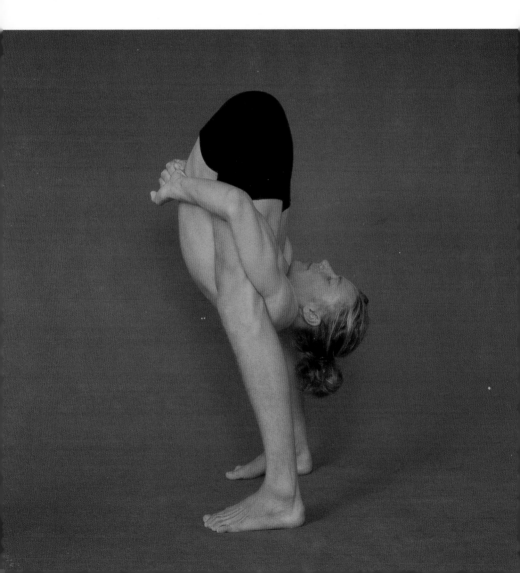

*Best way to learn*

No one is forced to learn yoga. You come to it. If it nourishes you, practise daily – traditionally six days a week with rest at the full moon and menstruation. Rest is a vital part of the yoga practice, too. Becoming obsessive about practising is to be avoided because that can be another form of grasping or attachment. We must learn to drink deep every moment of every posture and breath.

# The series

In Astanga there are three series of postures followed methodically step-by-step, linked with vinyasas (breath-connected movements). In each, the Suryanamaskara A and B (five each) and the standing foundation postures, demonstrated here, are followed, leading into the primary, intermediate or advanced series. The finishing postures and final breathing sequence consisting of inverted postures (shoulderstand and headstand) are always added to cool the body and mind towards final relaxation. A modified breathing sequence is shown here. Once you have learnt the series, you can practise anywhere – flat, hotel room, beach, office.

**1.** Primary series – Yoga Chikitsa. This means yoga therapy and the primary series, lasting one and a half hours, realigns the spine, detoxifies the body, builds strength, flexibility and stamina. Each posture leads to the next, artfully opening up the body and freeing the musculo-skeletal system. Regular practice calms the mind and brings ease of movement and proper alignment awareness.

**2.** Intermediate series – Nadi Shodana. This means nerve purification and the intermediate series cleanses the nadis or subtle nerves. The spine is made lithe and strong like a plant stem, with deeper backbends. A teacher may introduce a student to the intermediate series when the primary series is strong.

**3.** Advanced series – Sthira Bhaga. This translates as divine stability; sthira means steadiness or strength, and bhaga means good fortune, dignity. A handful of aspirants across the globe have achieved this awesome form, much of which is practised on the hands in arm balances.

# The method

Astanga Vinyasa yoga requires skill and endurance, involving an hour and a half of continuous linking postures. It is strenuous and does require a certain degree of fitness. Asanas are the same as those taught by B. K. S. Iyengar (see Chapter 2), but the difference is that Astanga Vinyasa links postures with vinyasas; the synchronized breathing movements, through a series. Having a set practice is hugely challenging because you have to find the resources inside yourself to follow the form: it is a wonderful, if rigorous, discipline.

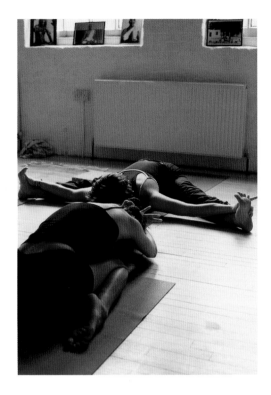

From the outside, an Astanga class will look intensely physical and quite acrobatic. This does not mean it is less spiritual. The body is cleansed and honed, and as you engage deeply in the physical, so also is the mind engaged, and emotional clearing takes place.

Although this method may appear to be focused on the Third and Fourth Limbs (asana and pranayama), Astanga Vinyasa yoga in fact synthesizes all the Eight Limbs of yoga in the moment, on the mat: they manifest through focus and intent. Practice is meditation, going directly to the unconscious and "feeling" parts of ourselves. Andy Levien, sound recordist, has practised advanced series intensively: "I think the practice is intense enough to not really need much more – because it is a meditation…on a good day."

## Pranayama

Concentrating on breathing slowly and deeply soothes the mind and nourishes the body with healthy blood and fresh oxygen. Breathing combined with flowing asanas eases tension in the body and mind. Breathing deeply also removes the limitations of fear and anxiety. For millennia ancient seers have employed the breath as a key tool to focus and concentrate the mind, leading towards stillness.

Ujjayi, deep thoracic breathing, involves partially closing the glottis with jalandhara bandha, giving a feeling of the breath filling the space between the throat and the heart with a sibilant sound reminiscent of scuba diving. The chest expands, developing strong, healthy lungs. Ujjayi breathing produces heat and destroys phlegm, and the Bihar School advises its practice in winter.

## Bandhas

The use of bandhas, the locks or grips that control vital energy in the body, is an advanced and evolving practice. Uddiyana bandha strengthens the lower back and helps us to move from the core of the body, safely and instinctively, rather than from the outer body. Uddiyana creates internal heat; the breathing releases toxins, purifying the body and letting healthy blood flow through.

## Suryanamaskars

Sun salutations form the opening sequence in Astanga Vinyasa yoga. They cultivate concentration, a deep focus, positive intention and proper alignment. They build up heat and sweat to detoxify the body, warming it up so you can stretch safely into deep postures.

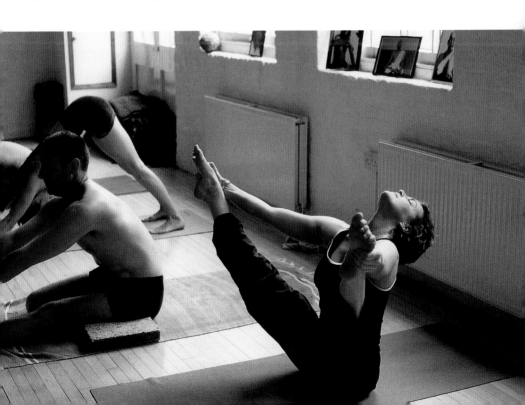

# Practice

Practice according to your fitness and do not try to rush. The aim is to develop a fluid sequence of asanas joined together with an unbroken thread of deep breathing to bring about a state of meditation in movement. Concentrating on the alignment and positioning of your body, you will be completely engaged and focused in the moment through the quiet, cleansing mantra of the breath. Asanas are held for five to eight breaths, which allows meditation through concentration on body, breath and gaze (drishti). Once the sequence is learned, you can enter deeper into the practice and observe mental fluctuations and emerging emotions. As we practise, we draw closer to ourselves. "Samskara" (conditioned patterns of behaviour) can be seen more clearly, and little by little released or accepted.

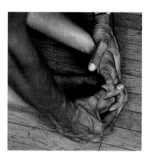

The teacher guides beginners through the elements of the practice. Like learning to swim, the student can gradually begin to venture out alone, having learnt the series (primary, intermediate or advanced). This can be daunting at first, and rightly so, because Astanga yoga is a discipline to help you on the continuous journey to self-mastery and integration. The teacher makes adjustments and coaxes the student into deep postures. It is essential to learn good alignment awareness from the start and it can be beneficial to attend Iyengar classes first.

Although this is a personal practice, to be explored alone, the shared energy of an Astanga class can be exhilarating and beautiful. In intense series, a class can become very hot.

By practising without a teacher, you are able to listen to the breath and can be more aware of thoughts passing through the mind like a filmstrip. The aim is to become detached from the drama, looking with deeper vision. This is pratyahara, sense withdrawal.

The half-hour programme presented here introduces the foundation practice of Astanga Vinyasa. To begin, there are two Suryanamaskar sequences, A and B. (See modifications if you suffer from a stiff back or other similar problems.) Suryanamaskar A consists of ten movements, which stretch and awaken the spine; Suryanamaskar B is a fluid, seamless sequence with deep breathing. B is a development of A but adds two new postures: Utkatasana (the Fierce posture) and Virabhadrasana (the Warrior pose). These two work on the alignment of the hips. They stretch and tone the body in artful sculpting, and cultivate concentration.

The two Suryanamaskar sequences are followed by standing postures which always progress in the same order. The final phase consists of breathing exercises before relaxation.

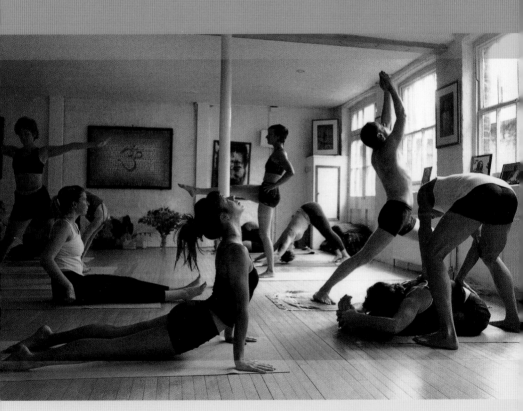

" **Practise**, practise, all is **coming**. " PATTABHI JOIS

# Suryanamaskar A

While learning the following sequence, take five breaths in each posture, in order to attain a feeling of a deep stretch and alignment awareness. Do not rush. Keep breathing a conscious ujjayi breath. Once you have learned each posture, build up a continuous sequence, sustaining the Downward Dog only for five breaths. (If necessary, rest in the Cat or child's posture.) The pictures illustrate how the sequence flows through each posture in vinyasas, breath-connected movement.

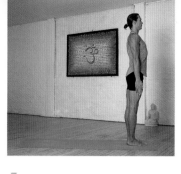

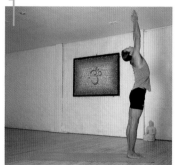

# Tadasana – Mountain Posture

Stand at the front of the mat, feet firmly grounded, legs straight. Lengthen the spine, lift the chest, gaze straight ahead and begin to breathe a soft, deep ujjayi breath by slightly narrowing the glottis at the back of the throat. The sound is sibilant, and the whole ribcage expands. Hollow the lower belly to protect the lower back and lift the perineum, the middle muscle in the pelvic floor. Keep your tailbone tucked down. You are harnessing three bandhas, breathing deeply and focusing.

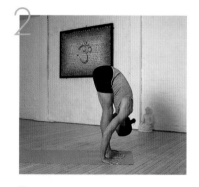

**1.** Inhale, raise your arms up sideways over your head. Press the palms together and look up to your thumbs. Your arms should reach up like an arrow.

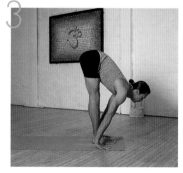

**2.** Uttanasana – Intense pose. Exhale, fold your body forwards, lengthening and releasing your spine. If possible, allow your abdomen to touch your thighs. Drop your head to lengthen your neck.

**3.** Urdhva Uttanasana. Inhale, look up, lift your chest and lengthen the wall of your abdomen. Place your hands beside your feet, with palms pressed down, fingers spread wide like a starfish.

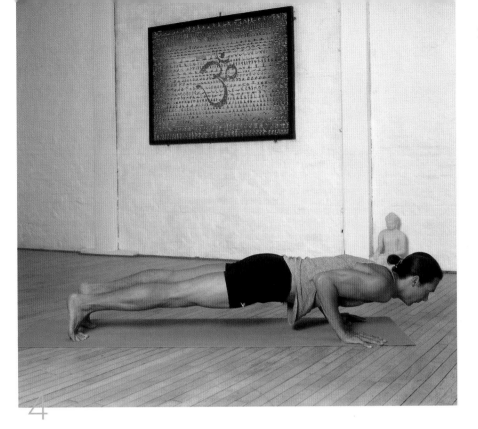

4

**4.** Chaturanga Dandasana – Four-angled Staff or Staff pose. Exhale, step or jump your feet back with your feet hip-width apart so you are in a straight plank position. Keep your back straight and strong in line with your legs. Your arms should be fully extended and your lower abdomen drawn inwards, creating a diagonal line through your body. Inhale, then exhale and gently lower your body to the floor, bending your elbows and pressing them into your side-ribs, while keeping your legs strong and straight. Your hands should be pressed, palms downwards, close beside your ribcage. (**Modification:** if this is too intense, lower your knees first, then your body. Do not strain your back.)

Tuck your toes under and press your palms deep into the mat beside your side-ribs. Making your body strong and straight, lift first your legs off the floor, then your abdomen, third your chest, creating a straight line. This may take some time and practice to achieve. If it is too hard, keep your chest touching the floor. Keep breathing!

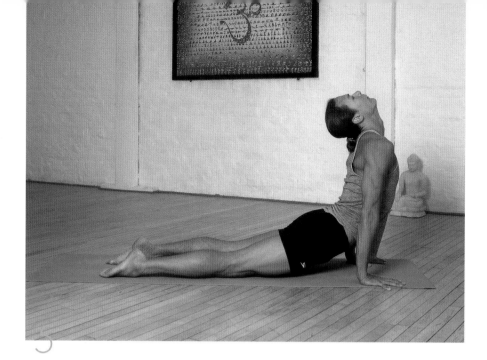

**5.** Urdhva Mukha Svanasana – Upward Dog. Inhale. If your toes are tucked under, roll over them, arching your spine. Look up, with only your hands and the tops of your feet touching the floor. Work your legs, squeezing the muscles, straighten your arms and broaden your chest.

(**Modification:** if this is too intense, keep your legs touching the floor, but strengthen them and arch your spine, keeping your elbows bent a little. Do not strain your back – strong legs should support the back.)

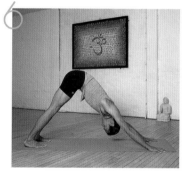

**6.** Ardho Mukha Svanasana – Downward Dog. Exhale, roll over your toes, pushing your hips up to the sky and pressing your heels towards the floor. Lengthen your spine, lift your front ribs away from your pelvis, hollowing your lower belly. Push away from your hands and straighten your legs. Press the palms of your hands down, especially the inside edges and stretch your fingers open like a starfish. Drop your chin to your chest to release your neck. Look towards your navel. Take five deep ujjayi breaths.

**7.** Inhale, bend your knees and look up.

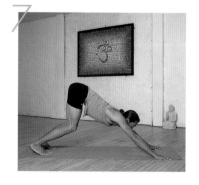

**8.** Jump or step your feet together between your hands, and exhale. Fold your head into your knees, releasing your spine. (**Modification:** if you have pain in your back, soften and bend your knees.)

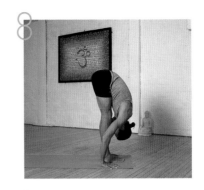

**9.** Raised Tadasana. Inhale, raise your arms in a sideways movement up over your head, press the palms of your hands together and look up.

**10.** Tadasana. Exhale and return your arms to the sides of your body.

Repeat the sequence five times until you can maintain the flow of breathing, so creating vinyasa, breath-synchronized movement, as well as building tapas (heat) and cultivating concentration. Always begin in the classical posture of Tadasana.

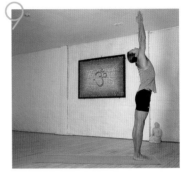

### Benefits

Suryanamaskar A concentrates the mind, making the body strong and flexible, shedding tension and stiffness.

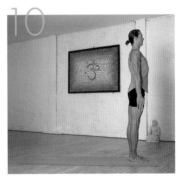

**"**It is only with the heart that one sees clearly.

What is essential is invisible to the eye.**"**

Antoine St Exupery, *The Little Prince*

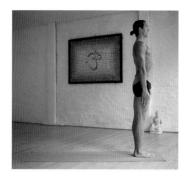

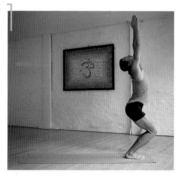

# Suryanamaskar B

The Fierce pose and the Warrior pose are now added. Suryanamaskar B moves through a flowing sequence based on Suryanamaskar A, so much of it will be familiar. Once you have looked at the flow of the movements, you can practise them by following the instructions for each in more detail. Make sure you keep your gaze (drishti) in the right direction.

Stand in Tadasana. Lengthen your spine upwards, breathing deeply. Ground your feet, press the inner seams of your legs together and lift the crown of your head. Draw your navel to your spine and lift the root lock, mula bandha.

**1.** Utkatasana – Fierce pose. Inhale, reach your arms up over your head, and drop your pelvis as if sitting into a chair. Gaze towards your thumbs, and hollow your lower belly.

**2.** Uttanasana – Intense pose. Exhale, and fold your body forwards out of your hips, keeping your knees soft as you release your spine over your thighs. Gaze towards the tip of your nose.

**3.** Inhale, lift your chest and look up, moving into Urdhva Uttanasana.

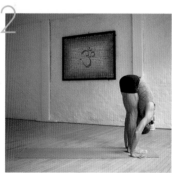

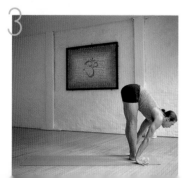

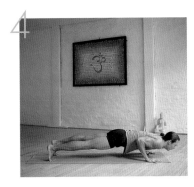

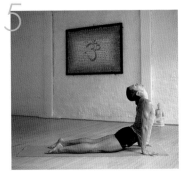

**4.** Chaturanga Dandasana. Exhale, lightly jump (or step) back and lower your chin into the Staff pose.
(**Modification:** if this is too intense, lie on the mat.)

**5.** Urdhva Mukha Svanasana -- Upward Dog. Inhale, roll over your toes, arch your spine and look up. (Rest your chest on the floor if necessary while you are learning.)

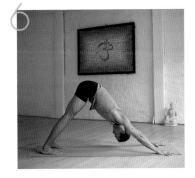

**6.** Ardho Mukha Svanasana – Downward Dog. Exhale and roll upwards over your toes pushing your hips back and pressing your heels to the floor. Gaze towards your navel. Take one full breath.

**7.** Virabhadrasana (first side) – Warrior pose. Inhale, pivot your left heel into your right big toe. Exhale and place your right foot between your hands.

Lift your upper body and bend into your right thigh, bringing your body parallel to the floor. Place your hands on your hips and, using your hands like a steering wheel, draw your right hip back and encourage your left hip forwards. Keep breathing as you align your body. Draw your stomach inwards between your front hip bones, and broaden across your chest. Share your weight equally between both legs as if you are sitting in a saddle.

Inhale, raise your arms over your head, press the palms of your hands together and look up. Lift your upper body out of your pelvis and lengthen your arms like an arrow.

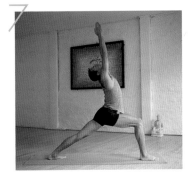

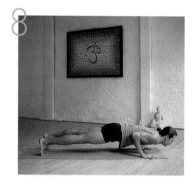

**8.** Chaturanga Dandasana. Exhale, lower your arms beside your front foot and jump (or step) back and lower your chin into the Staff pose. Empty your lungs.

**9.** Urdhva Mukha Svanasana – Upward Dog. Inhale, roll over your toes, arching your spine. Look up.

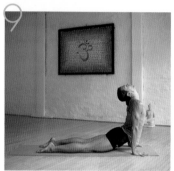

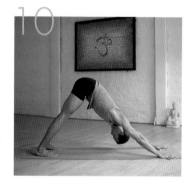

**10.** Ardho Mukha Svanasana – Downward Dog. Exhale, roll upwards over your toes, pushing your hips back and pressing your heels to the floor. Take one full breath.

**11.** Virabhadrasana (second side). Inhale, turn your right heel into your left big toe. Exhale, and place your left foot between your hands. Lift your upper body, bending deeply into your left thigh, bringing it parallel to the floor. Place your hands on your hips, encouraging the right hip to rotate forwards and the left hip to drop back. Inhale deeply into the bottom corners of your lungs and raise your arms over your head. Pressing your palms together, look up.

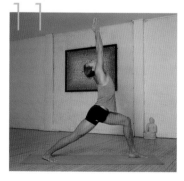

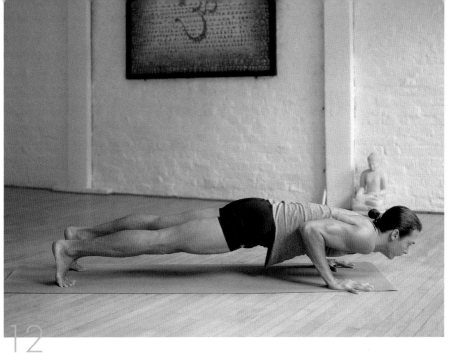

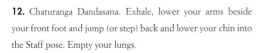

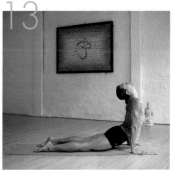

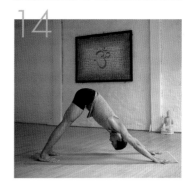

**12.** Chaturanga Dandasana. Exhale, lower your arms beside your front foot and jump (or step) back and lower your chin into the Staff pose. Empty your lungs.

**13.** Urdhva Mukha Svanasana. Inhale, roll over your toes into the Upward Dog, arching your spine.

**14.** Ardho Mukha Svanasana. Exhale, roll over your toes, press your hips back and lift your pubic bone. Press your heels down to stretch your hamstrings and calf muscles and take five deep breaths.

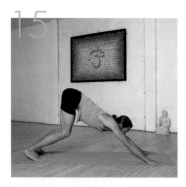

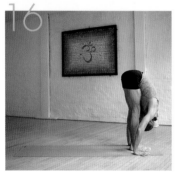

**15.** Inhale, bend your knees and look up, keeping your hips raised high.

**16.** Exhale, jump or step your feet between your hands and fold into Uttanasana, the deep forward bend.

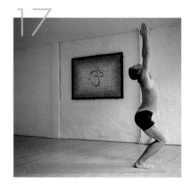

**17.** Utkatasana. Inhale, bend your knees, raise your arms over your head, gaze at your thumbs and press your palms together.

**18.** Exhale and release your arms, returning to Tadasana.

Repeat Suryanamaskar B five times, aiming to achieve an unbroken flow choreographed to the ujjayi breathing. If you are a beginner, repeat the sequence slowly, taking as many breaths as you need in order to find depth in each posture. Aim to build a sense of fluidity in your movements.

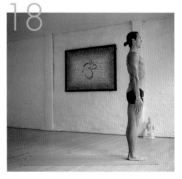

## Benefits

Uttanasana tones the liver, kidneys and stomach and can help alleviate period pain. It is also a good tonic for the heart and spine, and soothes the brain. Utkatasana unlocks the shoulders and develops the chest. It strengthens and aligns the legs, ankles and thighs, as well as toning the back, heart and abdominal organs. Chaturanga Dandasana, the Staff pose, tones the abdominal organs, and helps to strengthen the upper body and wrists. Urdhva Mukha Svanasana resembles a dog stretching. The whole of the front (east side) of the body is stretched, rejuvenating the spine, expanding the chest and opening the lungs. Healthy blood flows to the pelvic region.

Ardho Mukha Svanasana, the Downward Dog, stretches the whole of the back (west side) of the body, nourishing it and releasing the shoulders and neck. It is excellent for hamstrings, calves and the Achilles tendons. It strengthens the ankles and shapes the legs, while healthy blood flows to the torso and brain, slowing the heart.

Virabhadrasana, the Warrior pose, shapes, strengthens and tones the legs and back. It also massages the abdominal organs. Helping to realign the hips, this posture releases stiffness in the shoulders, back, ankles, knees and hips. It opens up the chest, encouraging deep breathing, and helps to slim hips and cultivate stability.

## Standing postures

The standing postures develop strength, flexibility and stamina. They powerfully realign the spine, balancing the left and right sides of the body, bringing flexibility to the hips, spine and shoulders. This sequence should take about 20 minutes.

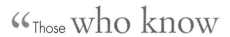

" Those who know do not speak. Those who speak do not know. "

LAO TZE

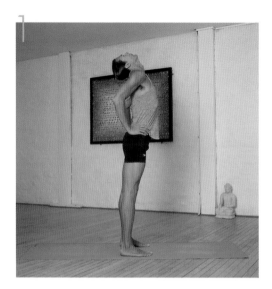

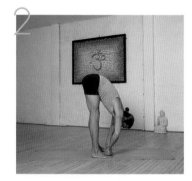

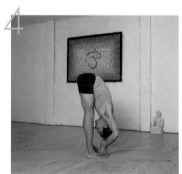

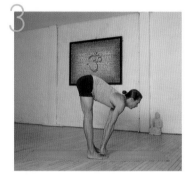

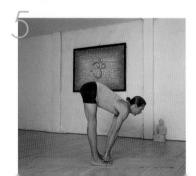

# Padangusthasana
– CATCHING THE TOES

**1.** Inhale, jump your feet hip-width apart. Place your hands on your hips. Exhale, spread your toes and square the outsides of your feet. Inhale, lift your chest and look up.

**2.** Exhale, fold your upper body from the front pelvis into a forward bend, catching the toes. The first two fingers should hook round the neck of the big toes.

**3.** Inhale, pull on your toes and look up, lengthening your abdomen and pulling it inwards.

**4.** Exhale, fold your body right over the thighs and release your spine into a forward bend. Take five ujjayi breaths. Breathe deeply and do not force your upper back or shoulders. Aim to touch your thighs with your abdomen. If necessary, keep your knees bent. Don't force your body or your breathing, but release your spine with every exhalation.

**5.** Inhale, lift your chest and look up.

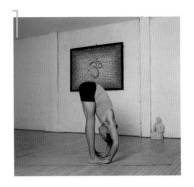

# Paddahastasana
## – STANDING ON THE HANDS
(padda means foot, hasta means hands)

**1.** Exhale and stand on your hands with your toes facing the inner part of your wrists.

**2.** Bend your knees to achieve the release of the lower back, if necessary. Inhale, lift your chest and look up.

**3.** Exhale, fold the body deeper, drawing your chin between your knees.

**4.** Breathe mindfully, balancing every inhalation with the corresponding exhalation.

**5.** Point your seat bones up and lengthen your spine with every exhalation. Take five ujjayi breaths.

**6.** Inhale, lift your chest and look up. Then exhale and place your hands on your hips. Draw your abdomen towards your spine and open your shoulders. Inhale, come up and look up.

**7.** Exhale, jump back into Tadasana, pressing your feet together. Take one full breath.

### Benefits
These postures help to tone the abdomen and spine, resting the internal organs and heart. They have a calming effect that helps to combat depression.

**"** ...if thine **own eye** be single,

the whole body shall be **full of light**. **"**

ST MATTHEW'S GOSPEL

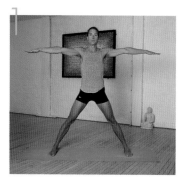

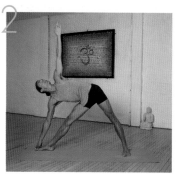

# Utthita Trikonasana
## – EXTENDED TRIANGLE

**1.** Inhale, jump to the right, so your feet land parallel, 3 feet apart. Exhale, lift your chest and roll back your shoulders.

**2.** Inhale, turn your left toes inwards 15 degrees, keeping your left outside heel grounded.

**3.** Exhale, rotate the ball of your right foot outwards 90 degrees. Draw back your left hip and ground your left foot. Inhale and lengthen your spine.

**4.** Exhale and tilt your body to the right, keeping your left hip and left shoulder drawn back.

**5.** Keep breathing and hook your right big toe with your right hand. If this is not possible, hold your right leg instead. Look up to your left thumb and open the palm of your hand. Keep your neck long, drawing your chin to your left shoulder (picture 2). Take five ujjayi breaths. Repeat the posture on the left side.

### Benefits

Twisting, nourishing and strengthening the spine, this posture also massages the internal organs and aids the elimination of waste matter. Ankles, knees, thighs are toned, the chest is developed, and the waist and hips slimmed.

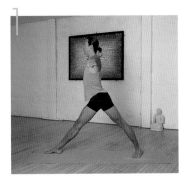

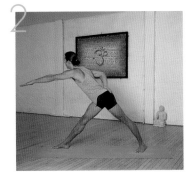

# Parivrtta Trikonasana
## – REVOLVED TRIANGLE

**1.** Inhale, press into the outer edge of your right foot as you come up from the extended triangle. Exhale and pivot your pelvis to the right. Facing over your right thigh, draw your right hip back.

**2.** Inhale and reach your left arm forward, stretching your left waist. Exhale and extend your upper body out of your pelvis, placing your left hand outside your right foot. If it doesn't reach, place your hand on your right leg. Inhale, place your right hand on your sacrum and twist your spine, drawing back your right shoulder and your right hip.

**3.** Exhale and extend your right arm to the sky. Look up to your thumb. Breathe deeply, lift your lower abdomen towards your spine, and tighten your leg muscles, keeping your legs strong and straight. Take five ujjayi breaths.

### Benefits

Twisting, nourishing and strengthening the spine, this posture also massages the internal organs and aids the elimination of waste matter. Ankles, knees and thighs are toned, the chest is developed, and the waist and hips slimmed.

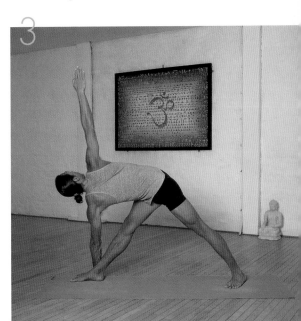

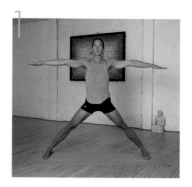

# Utthita Parsvakonasana
– EXTENDED SIDE-ANGLE

**1.** Inhale and jump to the right, gently landing with your feet about 4 feet apart. Your feet should be positioned beneath your wrists. Ground your feet and spread your toes. Exhale, roll back your shoulders and broaden across your chest, lengthening your spine. Inhale, turn your left foot in 15 degrees; exhale and turn your right foot out 90 degrees.

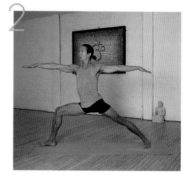

**2.** Inhale, draw back your left hip and ground your left foot. Exhale and bend your right leg deeply until your thigh is parallel to the floor. Root into your left foot, sharing equal weight between both legs. Inhale, lengthen your spine and broaden your chest. Exhale, keeping your left shoulder drawn back, place your right hand outside your right foot. Press your right knee into your armpit, creating a straight line between your right shinbone and your right arm. Inhale and raise your left arm over your head.

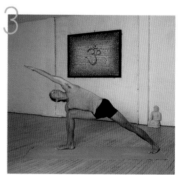

**3.** Exhale and extend your arm over your head, creating a diagonal stretch through the left side of your body. Breathe into your side-ribs and press the edge of your back foot down. Draw back your left shoulder and your left hip. Take five ujjayi breaths.

**Modification:** keeping your left shoulder open, place your right elbow on your right thigh. Draw your left hand behind you to catch your inner right thigh. Turn your chin to your left shoulder, broadening your chest. Open out the left side of your body as deeply as you can.

## Benefits

This posture gives a deep lateral stretch which shapes the waist and legs, tones the thighs, ankles and knees and develops the chest. It also aids the elimination of waste matter.

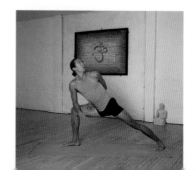

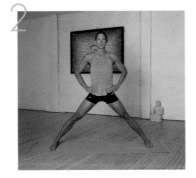

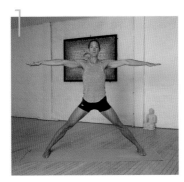

# Prasarita Padottanasana
– EXPANDED LEG (INTENSE STRETCH)

There are four variations of this posture.

## A

**1.** From Tadasana, bend your knees and, as you inhale, jump to the right with your feet parallel. Do not turn them outwards. Spread the balls of your feet wide and splay the toes. Ground your big-toe joints, the little toe edges, the inner and outer heels and tighten your leg muscles. Lengthen your spine and broaden your chest. Inhale and extend your arms out wide.

**2.** Exhale and place your hands on your hips.

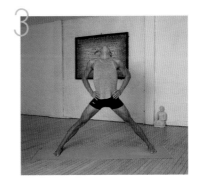

**3.** Inhale, lift your chest and look up.

**4.** Exhale and fold your body from your front pelvis, touching the floor with your hands. Place your hands in line with your feet and make sure your legs are wide enough to press your palms into the mat.

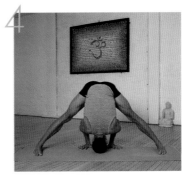

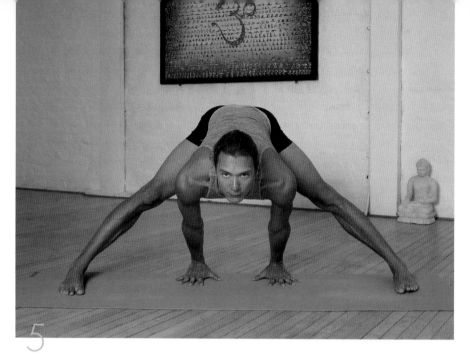

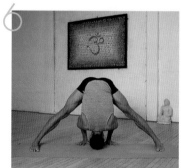

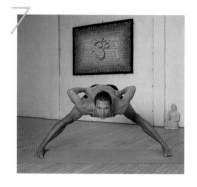

**5.** Inhale, look up and straighten your spine.

**6.** On the next exhalation, release into a forward bend again, breathing fully, and lift your front ribs away from your pelvis. Take five ujjayi breaths in this position.

**7.** Inhale and look up; exhale and place your hands on your hips, drawing your abdomen back towards your spine. Inhale and come up; exhale and release your hands to your sides.

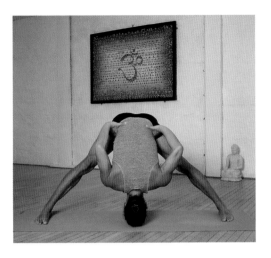

## B

**1.** From Tadasana, bend your knees and, as you inhale, jump to the right with your feet parallel. Proceed as for A.

**2.** Exhale and place your hands on your hips.

**3.** Inhale, lift your chest and look up.

**4.** Exhale and fold your body from your front pelvis, touching the floor with your hands. Place your hands in line with your feet and make sure your legs are wide enough to press your palms into the mat.

**5.** Inhale, lift your chest and look up.

**6.** Exhale, fold your body forwards from your front pelvis, keeping hands on hips, and bring your head to the floor (above left). Take five deep ujjayi breaths. Inhale, come all the way up, exhale and release your arms to your sides.

## C

**1.** From Tadasana, bend your knees and, as you inhale, jump to the right with your feet parallel. Proceed as for A.

**2.** Exhale and clasp your hands behind your back, interlocking your fingers.

**3.** Inhale, lift your chest and look up.

**4.** Exhale and fold your body forwards from your front pelvis, drawing your arms up over your head towards the floor behind you. Your palms should be facing into your body. Take five breaths, then sink your head down to the floor (right).

**5.** Inhale and come all the way up.

**6.** Exhale and release your arms to your sides.

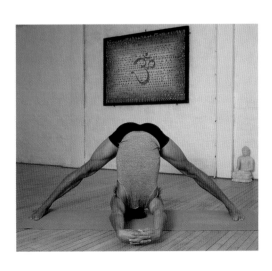

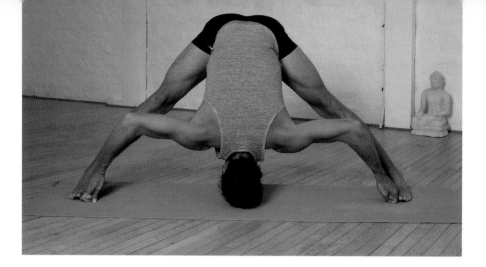

# D

**1.** From Tadasana, bend your knees and, as you inhale, jump to the right with your feet parallel. Proceed as for A.

**2.** Exhale and place your hands on your hips.

**3.** Inhale, lift your chest and look up.

**4.** Exhale and fold your body forwards from your front pelvis. Hook each big-toe joint with the first two fingers of each hand, with your palms facing in (above).

**5.** Inhale and pull on your toes, lift your chest and look up.

**6.** Exhale and draw your body forwards, aiming to keep your abdomen long and your spine as straight as possible. Do not bow your thorax or tighten your shoulders. Take five breaths, and with every exhalation release your spine, widening the space between each vertebra.

**7.** Inhale and look up; exhale and place your hands on your hips.

**8.** Inhale and come all the way up; finally exhale, release your arms to your sides and jump your feet back to Tadasana. Focus your gaze straight ahead of you, ground your feet, and stretch up through the core of your body.

### Benefits

This sequence of standing postures strengthens the legs and opens hamstrings. Blood flows to the upper body and head, nourishing the brain. All the standing poses help to balance and reduce body weight.

# Parsvottanasana
## – INTENSE SIDE STRETCH

**1.** From Tadasana, inhale, bend your knees and jump to the right.

**2.** Exhale as you land with your feet 3 feet apart and your arms wide. Inhale and bring your arms behind you. Exhale and press your palms together in the reverse namaste prayer position, fingers pointing up and with the edges of your hands pressed into your spine. Keep your chest open and your shoulders drawn back.

**3.** Inhale and pivot the ball of your left foot inwards 15 degrees; then exhale and pivot the ball of your right foot outwards 90 degrees. Draw back your right hip, turning your pelvis to face over your right thigh. Keep your legs strong and your muscles drawn up (picture 1 below).

**4.** Inhale and lean back, lengthening the front of your body and opening your shoulders and chest.

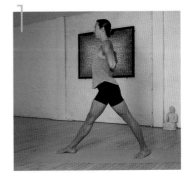

**5.** Exhale and extend forwards out of your hips, making a deep fold over your right thigh. Keep your spine long, lengthening your abdomen and drawing your navel to your spine. Drawing your chin to your shin, gaze at your big toe and ground your big-toe joint. Aim to align your spine over your extended leg. Draw back your shoulders and lift your chest. Take five ujjayi breaths, channelling your breath through the jalandhara bandha (picture 2 below).

**Modification:** if this strains your arms too much, fold your elbows behind your back instead.

### Benefits

This posture opens the hips, shoulders and wrists. The legs are made strong and supple, and the spine is awakened.

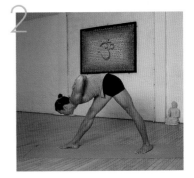

# Utthita Hasta Padangusthasana
## – EXTENDED HAND, FOOT AND BIG TOE

**1.** From Tadasana, root into your left foot, spreading your toes and tightening your left leg. Place your left hand on your left hip. Inhale and raise your right leg to catch either your shin or your big toe.

**2.** Aim to straighten both legs. The same principles of alignment apply – lift the upper body out of your pelvis, broaden across your chest and collarbones. Draw your navel in towards your spine and lift your pelvic floor. Take five ujjayi breaths.

**3.** Exhale, and with your raised right leg either bent or straight, open your hip, drawing your leg to the right, and turn your gaze to the left. Keep your spine long and stay strong in your back, drawing open your left shoulder. Take five ujjayi breaths.

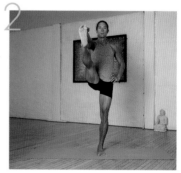

**4.** Inhale, bring your right leg back to the centre and hold on to your foot, ankle or heel with both hands. Exhale, centre your body and square your hips. Inhale and raise your right leg as high as you can. Keep your hips parallel.

**5.** Exhale and place your hands on your hips, and keep your right leg raised, pointing your toes. Use abdominal strength to support your back and your raised right leg. Sustain for five deep breaths, finding energy in your breath and bandhas. Exhale, release the position and realign in the Mountain pose.

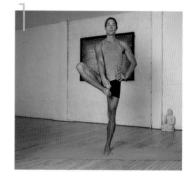

**Modification:** practise the posture with your knee bent, hugging your shin. Just take one breath in stages 3 and 4 of the leg raise. The alignment is of the utmost importance, not how high you raise your leg. Keep your back straight and balance the left and right sides of your body.

## Benefits
This posture shapes the legs and cultivates steadiness, balance and poise.

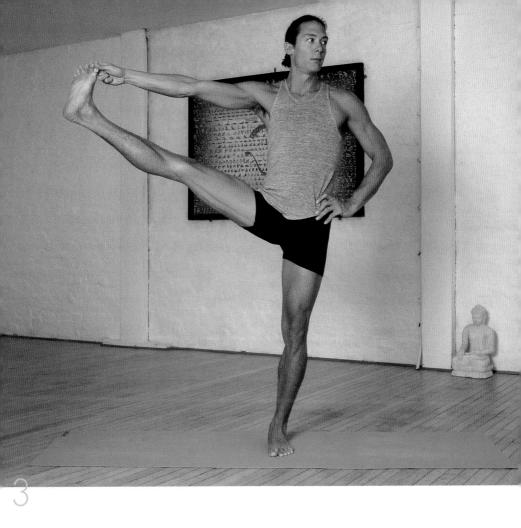

3

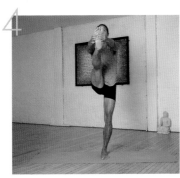

4

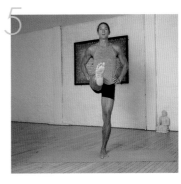

5

# Ardha Baddha Padmottanasana – TREE POSE

This sequence is the version that incorporates the half-lotus position. If you are attempting this posture for the first time, practise the version given under Modification (see below).

**1.** Ground your left foot and raise your right leg. Rotate your right hip as you drop your knee towards the floor, and bring your right heel high towards your navel.

**2.** Inhale and place your right foot into a half-lotus. Do not force your knee (see Modification). If you are an advanced yoga practitioner, bind the lotus by bringing your right hand behind your back and catching the big toe of your right foot.

**3.** Inhale and stretch your left arm upwards, keeping the crown of your head towards the sky.

**4.** Exhale and come forward, placing your left hand on the floor outside your left foot with your palm flat on the ground. Take five ujjayi breaths.

**5.** Inhale and look up; exhale and bend (soften) the standing knee.

**6.** Inhale and come all the way up; exhale, release your leg and return to Tadasana. **Modification:** press your right foot to your left inner thigh, as high as possible. Squeeze the muscles of the standing leg.

**7.** Draw your right knee as far back as possible and lengthen your spine. Place your hands into the namaste prayer position at chest level, then raise your arms like an arrow. Please do not strain your knees!

## Benefits

This posture tones and strengthens the legs, bringing balance and poise. The meditative quality of the balancing poses cultivates the "third eye" of intuition and inner vision.

This completes the foundation standing asanas, always practised in sequence, as presented here. The Warrior sequence and primary, secondary or advanced series would normally follow but this programme culminates in breathing sequences, leading into relaxation, as demonstrated by Matthew and Dominic.

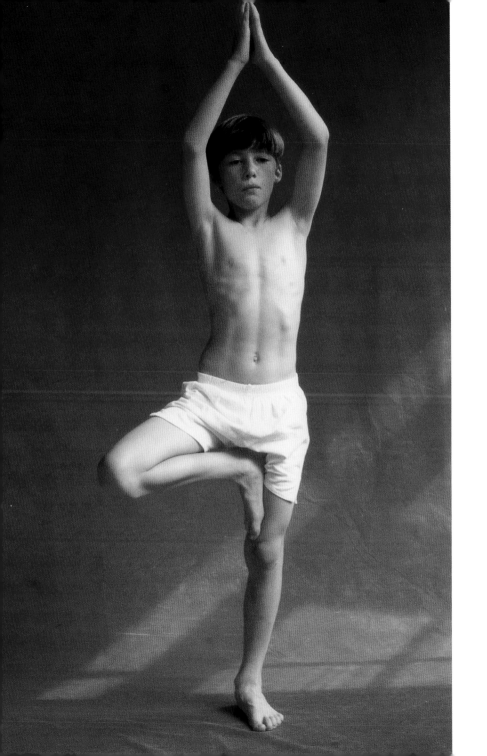

*"In all* **men** *there is the* eye of the soul, *which can be awakened by the correct means. It is far more* **precious** *than 10,000 physical eyes."* PLATO

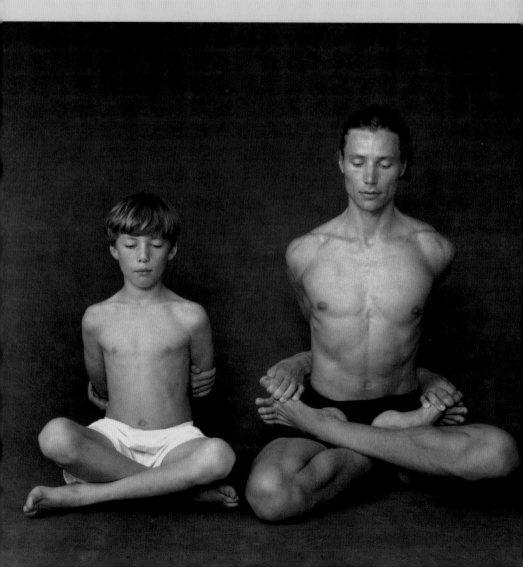

# Final breathing sequence

If you are comfortable in the Lotus posture with no strain on the knees, place the feet in Padmasana. If this is difficult, sit cross-legged.

Clasp your elbows behind your back and exhale into a forward bend. Take ten ujjayi breaths.

For advanced practitioners, reach your arms behind your back and aim to clasp your right big toe with your right hand and your left big toe with your left hand. Exhale into a forward bend. This is Yoga Mudra, Sealed Yoga posture. Take ten ujjayi breaths.

Inhale, return to centre, take 25 deep breaths, lower the eyelids and soften the mind.

### Relaxation – surrender

Lie in Savasana, Corpse pose, for 15 minutes.

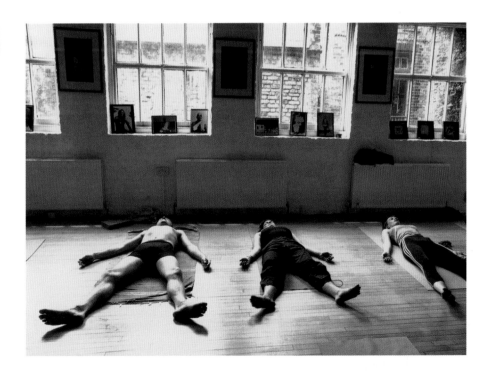

# Case Studies

Yoga teacher **MATTHEW VOLLMER**, semi-retired from civil engineering when he was 31. He describes Astanga Vinyasa practice as a long prayer: "It's an ever-changing thing – what it means to you is never the same, but I've seen a positive progression in the way I relate to myself and to others. When I started, I couldn't touch my toes. I didn't enjoy sport and I was all in my 'head'. My parents used to complain about my posture."

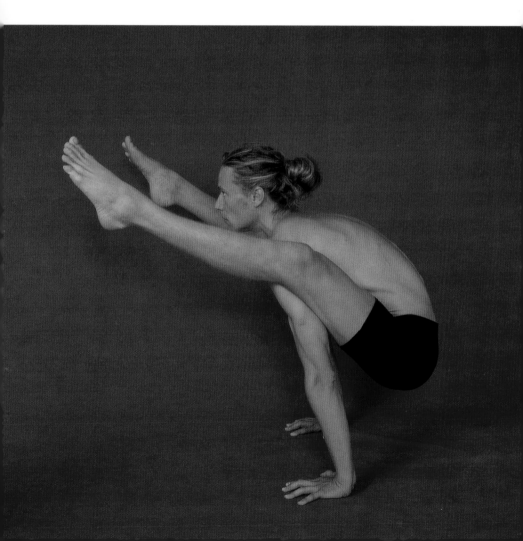

**LISSKULA**, originally a model, is currently finishing an MSc in work psychology. Like Matthew, she never enjoyed sport, but discovered Astanga Vinyasa yoga in 1997 and now practises it four mornings a week at 6 a.m. This is primarily for fitness, and she finds it difficult to define other reasons, but it is the one thing she enjoys, sticks to and feels like doing: "It carries me through the day. I don't feel good if I don't practise. It's such a thrill to make progress, to do headstands...I'd be devastated if I couldn't practise! It looks so beautiful, it can move me to tears." Lisskula began with back pain which has now gone.

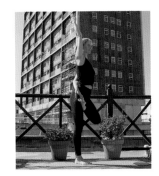

**CHRISTINA HATGIS**, an Astanga Vinyasa practitioner from New York, explains why she is so committed to this approach to yoga: "The repetition and the discipline keep me grounded in the moment. My thoughts can take me out of the moment into my head, and I lose the feeling of connection with my body. For me, the challenge of Astanga is to be on my mat and nowhere else for an hour and a half. It gives me that physicality which I love, and the moment."

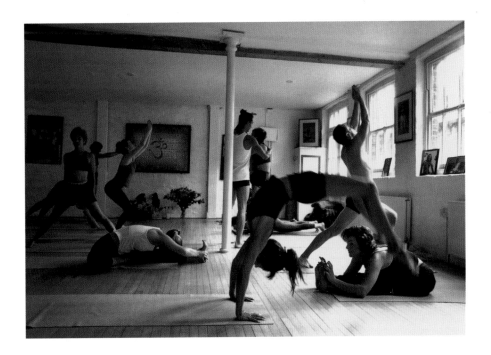

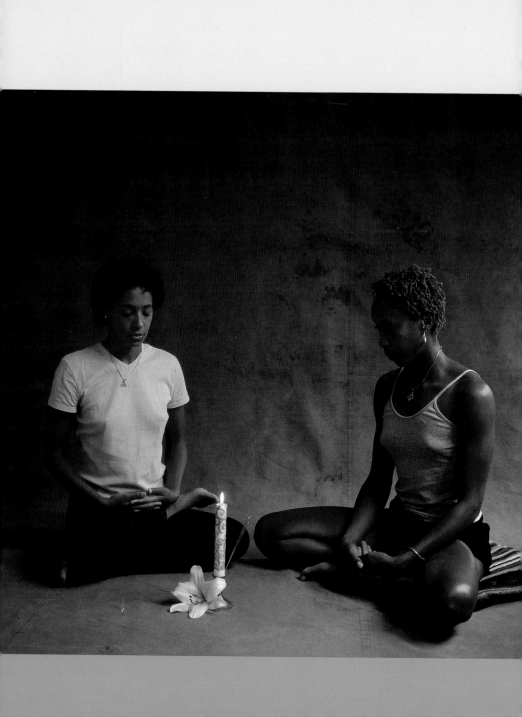

# SIVANANDA

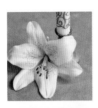

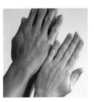

❝ There is only one caste, the caste of humanity. There is only one religion, the religion of love. There is only one language, the language of the heart . or the language of silence. Expand thy heart. ❞ SWAMI SIVANANDA

The Sivananda system is an integral system which involves five main principles: proper exercise (asana), proper breathing (pranayama), proper relaxation (savasana – physical, mental and spiritual), proper diet (sattvic – vegetarian food), positive thinking and meditation (dhyana, the Eighth Limb). Some practitioners take the view that Sivananda's gentle approach to asana tends to suit people who want to find relaxation through yoga, but it is accessible to everyone – all ages and all body types.

Various disciples of Swami Sivananda, including Swami Satyananda (see page 122) and Swami Vishnu Devananda, spread his ideas outside India in the 1960s. Swami Vishnu Devananda ("swamis" are Indian monks or "teachers who know themselves") studied under Swami Sivananda in Rishikesh for 12 years and came to the West in 1957, founding the International Sivananda Vedanta Yoga Centres. The first Sivananda teacher training course was established in 1969.

# Swami Sivananda

Born in 1887 in Madras State, southern India, Swami Sivananda came from a family of yogis. A karma yogi, he practised as a doctor in Malaysia for some years before discarding all material possessions to become a wandering mendicant. In 1924, at the age of 37, he returned to India and became a "sanyassin", renouncing the world and struggling with his spirit to follow the path of self-discipline and meditation. After one year, he settled in Rishikesh in the Himalayas, and for seven years immersed himself in intense spiritual practice. During this time he established a small medical clinic.

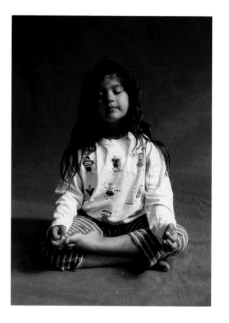

Swami Sivananda was aware of the emotional and mental suffering in the West, and the need to spiritualize daily life with the Eight Limbed approach to yoga to achieve self-mastery: "The only war worth fighting is the one within one's own mind." He stressed the importance of ahimsa (non-violence), bhakti (devotion, surrender) and karma yoga (service), setting the cornerstone of his philosophy in the words serve, give, love, purify, meditate, realize.

Sivananda recognized that the root causes of suffering are desire and attachment, which generate thought-waves like ripples in the mind and cloud clear vision. He advocated intuitive knowledge – bhakti knowledge – from the heart as opposed to the intellect: "Intuitive knowledge alone is the highest knowledge. It is the imperishable, infinite knowledge of truth. Without developing intuition, the intellectual man remains imperfect. Intellect has not got that power to get into the inner chamber of truth... Meditation leads to intuition."

In 1936 he formed the Divine Life Society, and went on to write over 300 books. He said, "The great book is within your heart. Open the pages of this inexhaustible book, the source of all knowledge. You will know everything."

# The method

In all the yogas the body is regarded as the container or vessel of the spirit; asanas clean the vessel, training body, mind and emotions. In Sivananda yoga, asanas are practised slowly to reduce production of lactic acid in the joints, although increased oxygen intake through deep abdominal breathing also helps to neutralize it. The method is systematic and structured.

### Pranayama

A Sivananda yoga class begins with two forms of pranayama (see page 126), developing an awareness of the breath and the mind before asanas are introduced.

### Suryanamaskars and asanas

After pranayama, sun salutations are practised to stretch and awaken the spine gently, rejuvenating the whole system. They are beautifully smooth, with just one step back at a time, contrasting with the jumps in the Astanga Vinyasa Suryanamaskars.

Twelve basic asana postures follow, and these should be mastered before adding more (there are said to be 84,000 in total!). Between asanas, rest in Savasana, Corpse pose. Even in a single class you are nourished by the simultaneous practice of exercise, relaxation and meditation.

It is interesting that the first two postures in the Sivananda sequence are headstand (Sirsasana), regarded as the "king" of asanas, and shoulderstand (Sarvangasana), the "queen" of asanas. Although they are difficult, the body has first been thoroughly warmed up with safe, stretching Suryanamaskars.

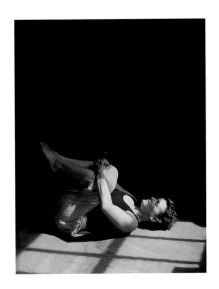

In Sivananda yoga the final two asanas consist of standing poses: Paddahastasana (standing forward bend) and Trikonasana (Triangle, lateral stretch). (In Astanga Vinyasa yoga these are included in the dynamic opening foundation sequence.)

As you will see, the Sivananda approach, which cultivates an overall feeling of integration and wholeness, is smooth, gentle and fluid, yet asanas can be practised in a way that suits all levels. Alignment is not emphasized in the same way as in Iyengar yoga, but postures are held for up to three minutes and should be comfortable.

## Bandhas

Bandhas and chakras (energy centres) can be incorporated in the second year when the practice is firm and strong.

## Karma yoga

Karma yoga is yoga of unconditional service and is suitable for active people. Satyananda stresses the value of interacting with the world, and describes how karma activity can be used to adjust samskaras (negative attitudes, mental conditioning) to bring balance. He said that our work should suit our abilities.

The *Bhagavad Gita* was written at the end of the Vedic period, approximately 600 BCE, shortly before the birth of Buddha, who, after years of searching, found enlightenment through meditating on suffering. A sublimely poetic Hindu text, the Mahabharata, its core, recounts a story of conflict between two sides of the same family, teaching about self-harmony, karma (service), jnana (knowledge) and bhakti (heart) yoga.

The main theme is of action combined with meditation. Krishna urges Arjuna to enter a yogic state in order to know the meaning of action within action – to be totally aware while acting with intense concentration. This principle runs through all the yogas.

# Swami Satyananda and the Bihar School of Yoga

Born in the Himalayan foothills, Satyananda encountered sages and saddhus – holy men – as a young boy, and they inspired him to continue his search for enlightenment. At the age of 19 he met his spiritual master, Sivananda, in Rishikesh. After 12 years immersed in karma yoga, Satyananda wandered extensively for nine years, practising yoga in seclusion and eventually coming to rest in Munger, by the River Ganges.

Here, in 1964, he founded the Bihar School of Yoga, which has become a focal point for yogic science, running its first teacher training course for Europeans in 1968. It was one of the first institutions to train female and foreign sannyassins, and to initiate women as well as men to become swamis. Now it has been made into a University, offering degree courses.

In 1998, Satyananda renounced the establishment, and began his life as a wandering saddhu.

A leading exponent of yoga and Tantra, Satyananda's dynamic and scientific approach has inspired and nourished spiritual seekers worldwide.

" The primary purpose of the practice of yoga should be to **integrate** the different planes of one's personality and at the same time to evolve the consciousness to gain greater knowledge of oneself. In this way any person anywhere in the world can fulfil his long cherished wish. "

SWAMI SIVANANDA

# Swami Pragyamurti

Swami Pragyamurti has been teaching since the 1960s. She came across the Bihar School of Yoga by chance and there, in 1969, met her guru, Swami Satyananda. Now based in London, she runs courses recognized by the British School of Yoga. She believes we need oases, sanctuaries for "the soothing and benevolent teachings of yoga", especially in cities, where there is tension and a concentration of poverty and separation between races and sexes.

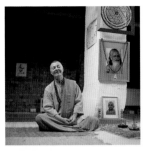

Swami Pragyamurti began yoga out of desperation – she was asthmatic, unhappy and restless. She fell in love with yoga's approach and style: "a way to be who you fully are and live a loving and useful life." For her yoga means oneness – "unity on all levels with the rest of creation."

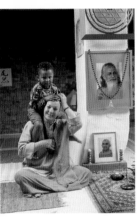

### Are Sivananda and Satyananda yoga suitable for everyone?
They won't suit people who don't want to change.

### Is it important to stay with one method?
It is better to concentrate deeply on one path.

### On egos
You can't be embodied without an ego. You need to make friends with it, not kill it, so you can avoid being a slave to it. Growing spiritually involves achieving a balance. You have to have it. You need to get in touch with your source of power and to become strong first. In meditation we watch the play of the ego. Within yoga systems we have the tools for transformation.

### On gurus
The guru shows light. The path isn't straight and there are many pitfalls. We cannot undertake a journey of this complexity without a teacher, if we are going to embark seriously upon it. You don't learn golf without a teacher.

### Best way to learn
Morning practice enables us to live as we want to: usefully, lovingly and interestingly. Practising in the morning cleans, prepares and aligns the body and mind to meet the challenges of the day.

**❝**An ounce of **practice** is worth several tons of **theory**.**❞** Swami Sivananda

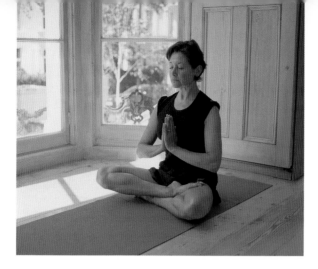

# The 12 Sivananda asanas

In Sivananda's ashram (retreat) in Rishikesh, 12 basic asanas are taught as a foundation for health. In his book *Yoga Asanas* he prescribes the headstand, shoulderstand and head-knee pose (as well as the Lotus posture) as "destroyers of diseases and bestowers of long life".

1. Sirsasana – headstand
2. Sarvangasana – shoulderstand
3. Halasana – plough; counterposture: Sethubandasana – Bridge
4. Matsyasana – Fish; counterposture to shoulderstand
5. Paschimothanasana – head–knee pose; counterposture: inclined plane
6. Bhujangasana – Cobra
7. Salabhasana – Locust
8. Dhanurasana – Bow
9. Ardha matsyendrasana – spinal twist
10. Kakasana – Crow (arm balance); Mayoorasana – Peacock
11. Paddahastasana – standing forward bend
12. Trikonasana – Triangle

Andrei Van Lysbeth is a Belgian yoga teacher who was one of the first Westerners to explore yoga in India (and possibly the first to experience Astanga Vinyasa yoga with Pattabhi Jois in Mysore). In his book *Yoga Self-Taught*, the headstand is placed at the end of the sequence with the shoulderstand at the beginning, so inverted poses begin and end the practice. Some people find this very beneficial because inversions bring energy and soothe the brain.

# Practice

This session covers three of the five Sivananda principles mentioned at the beginning of the chapter: pranayama, asana and savasana. The programme demonstrates opening pranayama exercises, a Suryanamaskar sequence and Savasana relaxation to finish. Meditation can be cultivated during practice. A vegetarian diet should be followed.

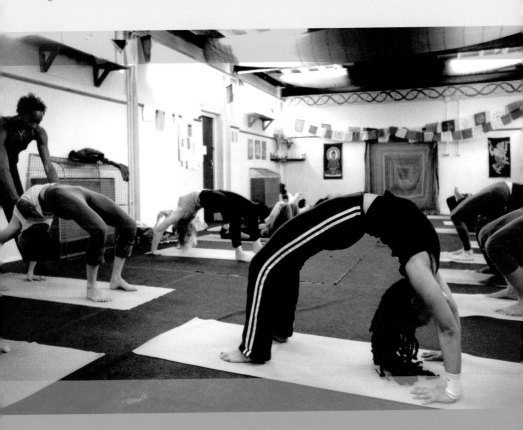

**❝** When my house **burned down,** I gained an **unobstructed view** of the **moonlit sky. ❞** Zen saying

> " It is of the **utmost importance** to concentrate the mind entirely upon the action of breathing... Air is our most **vital food**, and like any food it has to be digested, and this takes time. "

ANDREI VAN LYSBETH, *YOGA SELF-TAUGHT*

## Kapalabhati – CLEANSING BREATH

In this practice, which means "shining skull", a gentle, soft inhalation is followed by a sudden, strong exhalation. As you practise, it is important to keep the body as stable as possible, the shoulders and face relaxed.

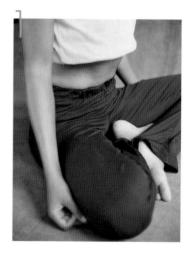

**1.** Sit comfortably with the back as straight as possible. Breathe freely, relaxing the abdominal muscles.

**2.** Make an gentle, soft inhalation through the nose, letting the abdomen fill out and expanding the lungs.

**3.** Exhale vigorously through the nose, pulling the abdominal muscles in and so pushing the air out of your lungs.

The following provides a safe framework, although it's best to learn with a teacher. Begin at the rate of one expulsion of breath per second. Increase to two expulsions per second. Start with ten expulsions only, every day for one week. In week two, practise one round of ten expulsions morning and evening; in week three, practise two rounds morning and evening. Gradually build up to 120 expulsions for each round.

### Benefits

This pranayama exercise cleanses the respiratory system, feeding oxygen to the lungs, strengthening them and draining the sinuses. Excess carbon dioxide is eliminated, which purifies the blood and increases prana (vital air) intake. The mind is invigorated, abdominal muscles strengthened, and liver, spleen, stomach and heart all massaged.

# Anuloma viloma
## – ALTERNATE NOSTRIL BREATHING

Sit as straight as possible, with seat bones grounded and chest opened out. Breathe freely. Make the gesture called Vishnu mudra by curling in the index and middle finger of the right hand so the thumb and fourth finger can be used on either side of the nose to close the nostrils.

**1.** Inhale through both nostrils.

**2.** Close the right nostril at the sinus bridge with the right thumb, exhale through the left nostril (right). Count to four.

**3.** Inhale through the left nostril while counting to four.

**4.** Close left nostril with the fourth finger of right hand, exhale through the right nostril, counting to four. Inhale through the right nostril counting to four (below right).

**5.** Close the right nostril, exhale through the left nostril counting to four. Inhale through the left nostril counting to four.

**6.** Release the right nostril and exhale completely.

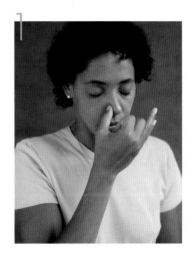

This is one sequence. You must first become comfortable with this breathing technique, then different ratios can be added, deepening the exhalations to twice the length of the inhalations – but you must learn this technique with a teacher. Retention of the inhalations can also be developed. Ten sequences are usually practised daily.

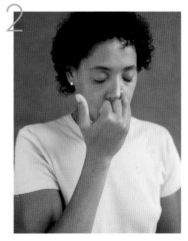

## Benefits

This pranayama also strengthens and purifies the lungs, purifies the nadis (energy channels) and increases prana intake. Stale air is eliminated, as you increase the length of exhalation; retention of inhalation increases oxygen intake. Stilling the breath stills the mind!

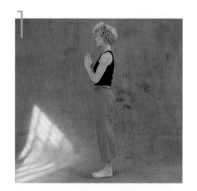

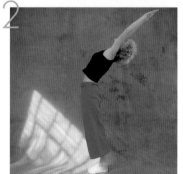

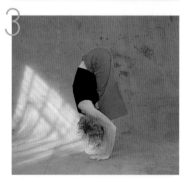

## Asanas

As taught by the Sivananda ashram in Rishikesh, the Suryanamaskars consist of 12 movements and can be practised by anyone at any age. Andrei Van Lysbeth, who describes them as a "splendid exercise" without which a yoga session is "inconceivable", suggests 15 rounds in five minutes.

**1.** Stand in Tadasana, Mountain posture, with feet together. Take a deep, full breath. Exhale and place your hands in namaste, the prayer position.

**2.** Inhale and stretch your arms up over your head, arching the spine. Look up.

**3.** Exhale and fold into a forward bend, placing your hands on the floor beside your feet.

**4.** Inhale and stretch the left foot back, placing the left knee on the floor. Look up.

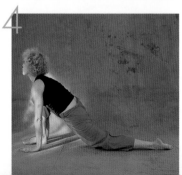

**5.** Holding the breath, bring the right leg back into "push-up" position, with both legs straight from head to heels, balancing on your toes.

**6.** Exhale, drop your knees to the floor, lower your chest to the floor between your hands, bending your arms, and lower your chin or forehead to the floor.

**7.** Inhale and slide the body forwards, arching your spine into the Cobra posture. Look up. (Legs and feet should be stretched out on the floor.)

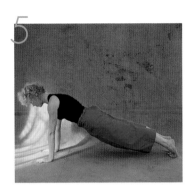

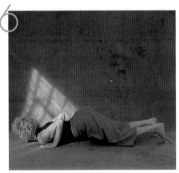

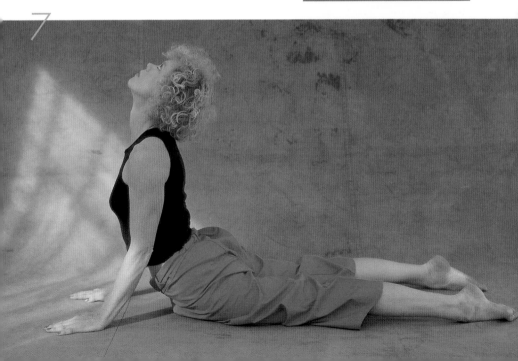

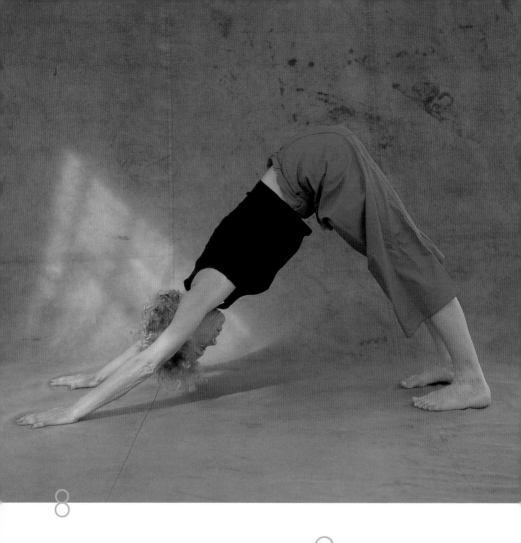

8

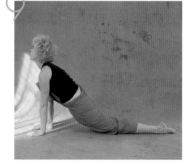

**8.** Exhale and push your hips back up to make the top of a pointed arch in a Downward Dog pose, dropping your head and stretching your heels down into the floor.

**9.** Inhale, bend your right leg to move your right foot forwards and place it between your hands, dropping the left knee to the floor (with left leg still stretched back). Look up.

**10.** Exhale and move the left foot forward next to the right foot. Fold yourself into a standing forward bend, head to knees.

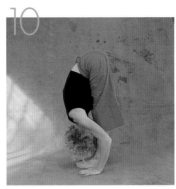

**11.** Inhale, stretch your arms over your head, look up and arch the spine.

**12.** Exhale, release your arms down to the sides of your body, and relax.

### Benefits

This sequence is a tonic for the whole system. As breath and movement are synchronized, the whole muscular structure is exercised, cardiac activity is increased, and blood flows better through system. The spine is awakened, internal organs massaged, digestion stimulated and constipation alleviated. The skin is refreshed, the mind is calmed.

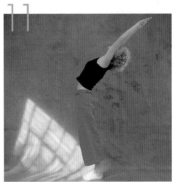

## Savasana

The closing, relaxing Corpse posture brings ease to muscles, nerves, mind and soul, as you absorb the effects of the asana practice.

**1.** Lie on your back on a firm surface, lengthening your spine, stretching your legs out from their hip sockets and your arms from the shoulder joints. Keep your feet quite close together, allowing them to fall open. Let your arms relax a little away from the body, palms turned upwards, fingers softly curling inwards.

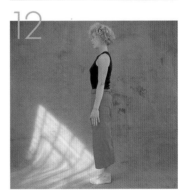

**2.** Nestle into the floor, particularly in the lumbar region and the back of the neck, as if nestling into warm sand. Close your eyes. Breathe slowly.

**3.** Relax all the muscles, nerves and organs in your body. Begin with your toes and slowly concentrate on each part of your body up to your head, face and brain. Repeat the mantra "om". Do not sleep, but meditate gently.

# Case Studies

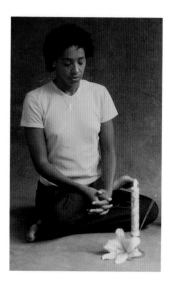

**SABEL** first learned yoga breathing as a young girl with her mother, because she was sleepwalking. She chose deep, abdominal yoga breathing rather than medicine to cure it. At 16, she did her first exercises, rolling to and fro on her back, felt electricity, and "that was it!"

"Anything you do in your adolescence stays with you. Your mind is like a CD-ROM, and when you do something deeply, it imprints deeply."

Through the 1980s Sabel immersed herself in yoga, attending Sivananda ashrams for a month every year.

"Ashram life is very structured. A day includes meditation, bhajans (reading from a spiritual book), devotion, asana practice (the twelve postures) and meals (vegetarian). At the end of the day you write in your spiritual journal because they say the mind forgets the lessons of the day."

**JUSTINE HARDY** is a writer, journalist and documentary maker, now qualified as a Sivananda teacher. In 1990, at the age of 24, she was attracted to the holistic and all-encompassing feel of Sivananda and started practising this method of yoga at the Sivananda ashram in Kerala, southern India.

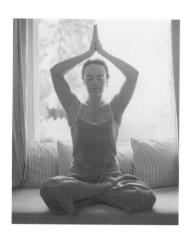

"Yoga is such a powerful journey to start out on. It is also a very personal journey into the truth of what lies beneath the layers we build up over our lies."

Justine regards Sivananda as an excellent introduction to yoga because it is gentle and presents a clearly defined lifestyle encompassing breathing, posture, service, devotion and diet. She believes in the path of yoga and that different styles suit different personalities. She varies her practice with Astanga Vinyasa yoga.

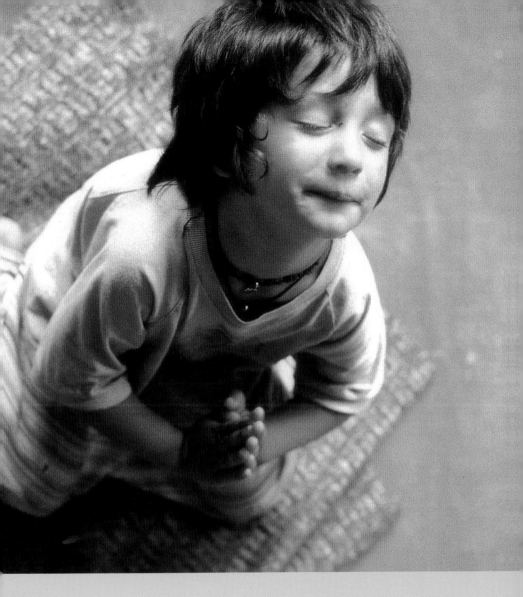

"Without going out of doors, one may know the entire universe: without looking out of the window, one may see the way of heaven. The further one travels, the less one may know. Thus it is that without moving you shall know; without looking you shall see; without doing you shall attain." LAO TZE, *TAO TE CHING*

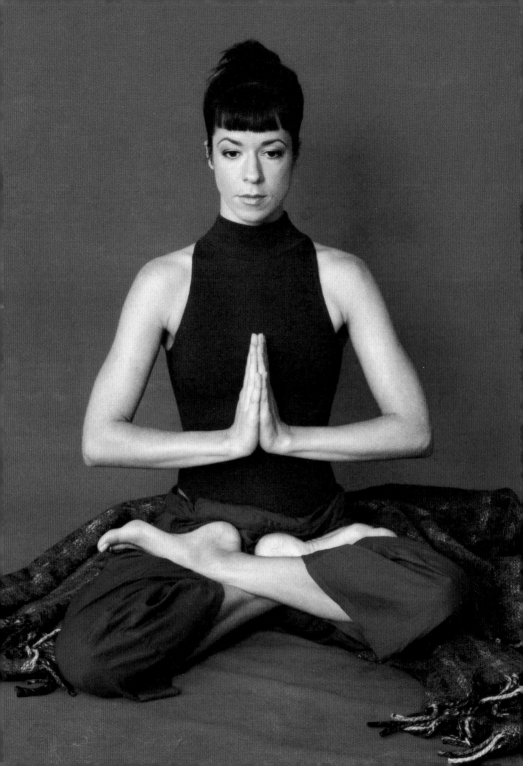

# TANTRA

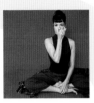

" This world is a manifestation of spirit.

Matter is spirit cognised through the senses.

Matter is spirit in manifestation. Matter is

spirit in motion... The fundamental error of all

ages is the belief that the spiritual world

and the material world are separate. "

Georg Feuerstein

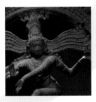

Tantra, "the cult of the feminine", is the root of yoga and the most all-inclusive spiritual system ever developed. Yoga is well known whereas Tantra is shrouded in mystery, yet, Swami Satyananda said, "Tantra is the mother, yoga is the son." The word itself is made up of two parts: "tanoti" meaning to expand, stretch or extend, and "trayati" to liberate or to free.

This bold philosophy concerns expanding your awareness of everything, and is described by the Bihar School of Yoga as a universal, practical system for diverse cultures throughout the world to engender higher awareness and spiritual insight. It encompasses a vast range of topics and all aspects of life and its origins reach far back into prehistory.

Tantra does not sit comfortably with dogma; it is not locked into a fixed view of the universe. Even its texts have changed and evolved over time, and the exact source of Tantra cannot be traced. Swami Pragyamurti says that Tantra started with the first human being, and is as old as time: "The Tantric attitude is wonderful because it allows you to start with what you are, here and now, without judging. It is non-dogmatic."

Straddling Hinduism and Buddhism, both defined by the concept of continuity, Tantra appeared in the opening centuries of the first millennium (of the Christian era). Original Hindu Tantric texts number at least 64, but few have been translated into European languages. They are presented in dialogue form and attributed to a divine rather than human author. Each includes discussion on the creation, the history of the world, male and female deities, ritual worship, especially of goddesses, Ayurveda (classical Indian medicine – see page 37), astrology, the subtle body, the nature of enlightenment and sacred sexuality.

## Arthur Avalon

Driven to protect the Tantras, Sir John Woodroffe, a judge of the Indian High Court in Calcutta in the last decade of the nineteenth century, devoted his personal life to dispelling prejudice by publishing and writing Tantric texts under the pseudonym of Arthur Avalon. Trying to win over his judgmental readership, he emphasized that Tantric practices are for adepts who have conquered desire and transcended any attachment to sensory pleasures. He went to great lengths to preserve and validate the texts.

Many Tantric texts were written in symbolic "twilight language" which shrouds them in secrecy so that they can be deciphered only with the guidance of an initiated guru – a way of protecting them from misuse. A guru is therefore essential to follow the razor-edged path of Tantric training.

" How can you turn your back on the divine creation? How can you dissociate the spiritual from the material? " SWAMI PRAGYAMURTI

# Anchoring spirituality in the mud of life

Yogis and quantum physicists share a wonderful view of the universe as a sea of "quantum foam", of space and time existing not as fixed realities but as mental constructs. The yogi is concerned with the unseen, the metaphysical beyond the world of manifested reality, and seeks union with this "unspeakable mystery". Tantra perceives the two realities of the seen and the unseen as inseparable, viewing the world like the warp and weft of a fabric, equally interweaving the material with the spiritual, regarding both as equal.

The subtle, non-physical world can be perceived through training in higher states of awareness, or what twentieth-century mystic Evelyn Underhill describes as "mystical perception".

Yoga and Tantric practice train us to open up the inner world. Hatha yoga expresses the ideal of Tantra, essentially finding bliss by anchoring spirituality in the "mud of life" rather than by withdrawing from it. Tantra anchors spirituality in real life, not in some celestial place. It roots spirit to earth, in the body, and celebrates it.

# Harnessing the energy of desire

Tantra embraces everything, including sexual energy, one of the most powerful energies in the body, powerful enough to create new life. Harnessing it and redirecting it around the body is an extremely effective way of energizing oneself. This makes Tantra radical, for it employs the physical as a path to ecstasy. The essence of Tantra is dealing skilfully with pleasure, using the energy of desire as fuel for spiritual awakening.

The radical view of the body being of equal importance to the mind in its training makes Tantra and its practices open to controversy and speculation. Widely misunderstood and often confused with Hindu erotic arts (kama shashtra), Tantric sexual practices are just one facet of a vast system and are enacted in only one school, though understood symbolically by others. However, Tantra today is held in low esteem in India, and the gatherings that involve sacred sex are suppressed by the Indian government.

"Longing is the fountainhead of ecstasy." KAHLIL GIBRAN

# Shiva and Shakti

Tantra dynamically views the universe as an ecstatic dance, and the body is part of this dance. Indian Tantra consists of two aspects: the male Shiva, signifying consciousness, and the female Shakti, symbolizing transformation.

Shiva, the foremost among yogis, is portrayed as the primeval lord of dance and destruction, an image that has fascinated physicists. The classical Hindu image of Nata-Raja, Lord of Dance, is described by Georg Feuerstein as the master weaver of time and space, who dances out the rhythms of the universe in cycles of creation and destruction: "The friend of outcastes, and hung with snakes, he finds reincarnations for lost souls, haunting cemeteries, holding poison in his throat. He is smeared with the ashes of destruction – all that life may come anew, and he embraces the most shunned of reptiles."

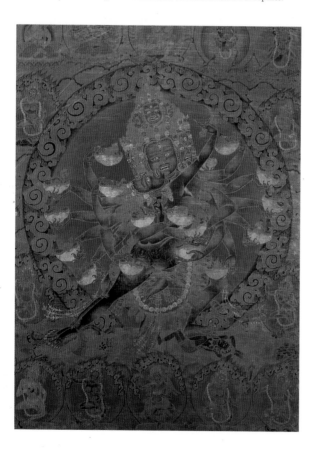

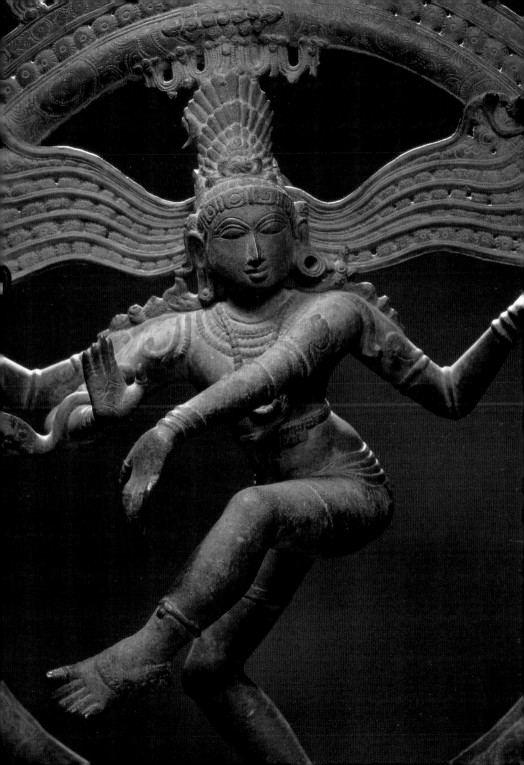

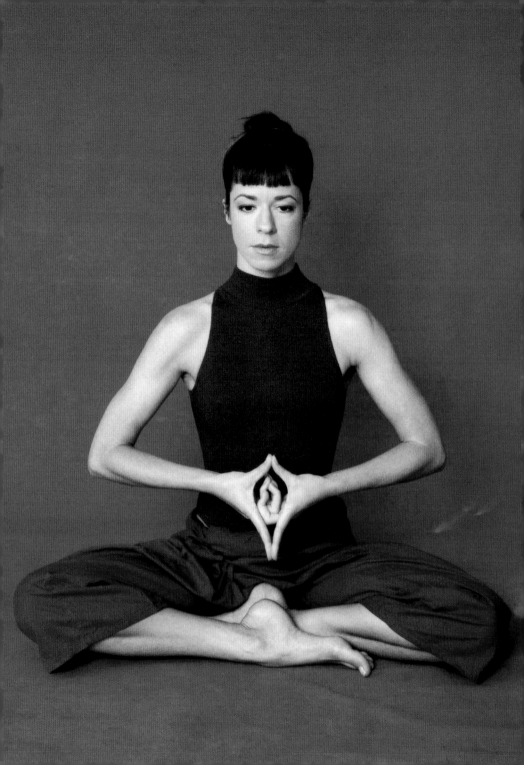

According to Tantra, every man and woman encompasses a complete union of universal energy, and everything we need in order to be complete is within us. Fundamentally, our deep essential nature is pure and clear, and the basis of spiritual practice is to remove the layers that cloud it. This innocence, that of a newborn baby, is the vision that we seek to recover.

Goddess worship thrived in ancient Vedic times and is central to many Tantric schools. Shakti, regarded as the cosmic mother, or mother nature, represents the feminine principle of universal creative energy, and is the driving force that brings transformation. Shakti embodies what psychologist Carl Jung called the "anima", the feminine psychic principle. She symbolizes the latent vital energy in the body stored as a snake (kundalini), coiled at the base of the spine. If awakened through yoga, she symbolically rises to unite with her spouse Shiva in sahasrara, the top chakra (energy centre) situated at the crown of the head.

One of the key yoga texts, the *Hatha Yoga Pradipika*, presents this concept of the divine embrace between Shiva and Shakti as a symbol of cosmic union, where self-identity (ego) and separateness disappear, where Shiva (formless, the unmanifest) and Shakti (form, the manifest) signify the two aspects of infinite reality. Their embrace is an archetype for the union of body and mind.

## Yin and yang

Tantra differentiates two main groups of people who are predominantly "yin" or "yang" by nature. Yang characterizes those who are extrovert, masculine and dynamic, predisposed to the path of activity and sensual enjoyment. Yin characterizes people who are receptive, feminine and passive. Those who follow the path of introversion, looking inward to know the real self. There are Tantra practices for both groups of people, but it is the yin aspect, the path of introspection, that is thought more likely to lead to bliss.

" He who knows both vidya (the inner world) and avidya (the outer world) crosses the abyss of death through avidya and attains immortality through vidya. " *ISHAVASYA UPANISHAD, VERSE 11*

# The method

As well as the pranayama, asanas and Suryanamaskara common to other approaches, Tantra employs mystical symbols and sacred sounds from the language of rituals, to give a map to navigate the inner world. We are entering a subtle, impalpable realm and need a different way of listening and seeing. Mantras, yantras and mandalas are vehicles to carry us into the beyond. All spiritual systems employ symbols.

### Mantras

Mantras – subtle sound structures and sacred phrases – bring liberation through inner resonance. Focusing on a mantra leads consciousness towards an inner perception of the "primal vibration" – "nadabindu", meaning literally "seed sound emanated from the universe".

Repetition of a sound phrase creates a wave pattern, called "japa", thus providing a device for mental penetration, much like the absorbing experience of singing plainsong or Gregorian chant. As well as achieving inner resonance through sound vibration, breathing is controlled, and the effect can be deeply meditative.

The highest reaches of subtle sound are embodied in the mantra "om"; the physical symbol is the conch shell. The effect of attaining the peak of om repetition is described as tranquil, soundless, fearless, beyond sorrow, blissful, immovable.

### Yantras

Whereas mantras work through sound resonances, yantras work through the organization of visual patterns. A yantra is a mystical symbol of cosmic energies and powers which acts as an instrument to induce meditation as you concentrate on it. It is a geometric diagram typically consisting of circles, lotus petals, triangles and sometimes deities. Contemplation is focused on the centre point or "bindu", considered to be the sacred symbol of the universe.

Yantras are concerned with looking beyond appearances to penetrate into the structure and essence of a thing; the understanding of a yantra grows gradually.

### Mandalas

More pictorial than a yantra, a mandala is based on a circular arrangement of complex patterns and iconographic images. Mandalas and yantras influenced the ground plans of Hindu and Buddhist temples. Stonehenge in southern England and the Mayan pyramids in Mexico are also examples.

> " With the body, head and neck held upright, direct your awareness to the heart region; and then 'AUM' will be your boat to cross the river of fear. "
>
> *Svetasvatara Upanishad*

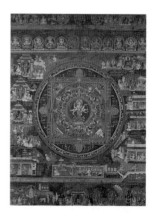

Much discussed by Carl Jung as a therapeutic art form, a mandala represents the integrated personality, symbolizing psychic unity that the subconscious mind can recognize.

Each person is a mandala, every thought is a mandala, and sexual union is a mandala.

## Mudras

The gestures that we make have an effect on us. Originating from the symbolic hand gestures of Indian dancing and Hindu rituals, mudras concentrate and channel energy flow in the body. There are said to be 108 mudras altogether. The universal mudra is "namaste", the prayer position, which transcends all boundaries.

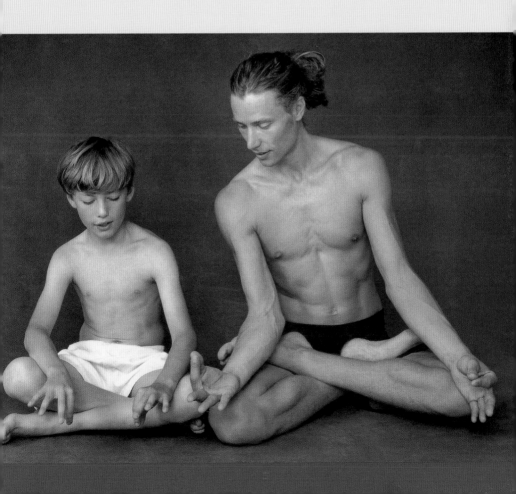

# Practice

Hatha yoga exercises are an important part of Tantra and stimulate release of inner energy, kundalini. As mentioned earlier, the path of Tantra requires careful guidance from a guru. In preparation, however, beginners can practise the following short sequence, as outlined by the Bihar School of Yoga. The importance of Paschimottanasana, the soothing seated forward bend which encourages introspection, is emphasized; and karma yoga is also of central importance. Hand mudras and yantras are much valued, including gazing on the shree yantra. Meditation is kept as simple as possible, avoiding complex techniques. Pranayama techniques, with breath retention and different breathing ratios, are taught by a qualified teacher. The key is regular practice.

## Suryanamaskars

Sun salutations are taught in the Rishikesh style (see pages 128–31). These should take five minutes.

### Savasana – CORPSE POSTURE

**1.** Lie supine, arms by the sides of your body, palms facing upwards. Legs should be straight and slightly separated.

**2.** Close your eyes and feel the parts of your body that are in contact with the floor. This develops awareness of the different parts of your body. Breathe freely. Be aware of your whole body sinking into the floor.

Savasana should be practised whenever you feel tired or tense. Wear enough to keep warm in this posture.

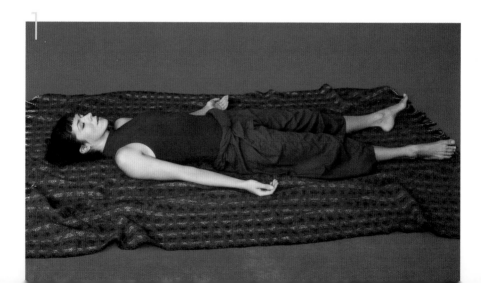

# Bhujangasana

This asana emulates a cobra rising up to strike its prey.

**1.** Lie on your front, legs straight with soles of the feet uppermost.

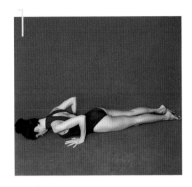

**2.** Place the palms of your hands on the floor vertically below but slightly to one side of the shoulders. Bend your elbows so they point backwards. Rest your forehead on the ground, and relax your whole body, especially the lower back (picture 1).

**3.** Inhaling, draw up the top half of your body, starting from the head. Now lift head and shoulders right off the ground (try to keep your navel in contact with it), begin to press your hands into the mat, and straighten your arms. Arch the spine without strain. Keep your arms and legs as relaxed as possible. Straighten your arms according to the flexibility of your back and use low synchronized movements linked with each breath (pictures 2, 3 and 4).

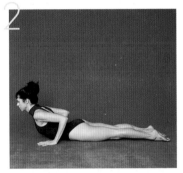

**4.** Exhale and lower yourself to rest your forehead on the ground, relaxing the whole body.

Repeat the movement a number of times. Do not strain. Listen to your body and your breath.

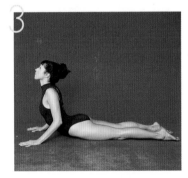

## Benefits

This posture makes the back flexible, stimulating the spine, which sends nervous impulses from the brain to the body. The pelvic region and internal organs are massaged and toned, compressing the kidneys which purify the blood. By broadening the chest deep breathing is encouraged and anxieties calmed.

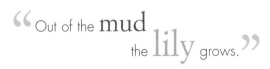

" Out of the mud the lily grows. "

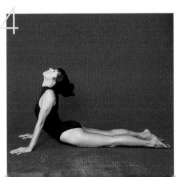

# Paschimottanasana

The seated forward bend is known as "tuning the west". The west refers to the back of the body and the front of the body is referred to as the east. "Uttan" means to stretch. This is a powerful asana, stimulating the central nadis (energy lines) in the spine.

**1.** From a seated posture, with legs straight out in front, place your hands on your knees, palms facing downwards. Relax the body, especially the back muscles.

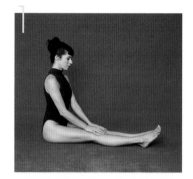

**2.** Inhale deeply, then, as you exhale, gently fold your trunk forwards, sliding your hands down your legs. Do not strain, but aim to reach far enough to catch your toes. Consciously relax your back. Keep your legs straight, exhale a little further into the posture.

**3.** Eventually you are aiming to lower your chest and abdomen on to your thighs, but it's a progressive exercise, so do not strain. Close your eyes.

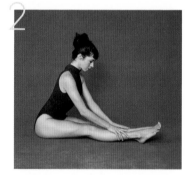

**4.** Inhaling, ease out of the pose.

## Benefits

The benefits of this asana cannot be overemphasized, as stated in the *Hatha Yoga Pradipika*: "Principle among asanas, Paschimottanasana causes vital energy to be carried up the spine. As well, it stimulates the digestive fire, slenderness in the abdomen and freedom from sickness for all."

Practise for as long as is comfortable. You may wish to repeat the posture three times.

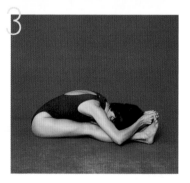

# Ardha Matsyendrasana

The half spinal twist is named after Yogi Matsyendranath, who meditated in this asana. A beautiful Hindu myth explains its origins. It is said that Lord Shiva, wishing to bring yoga out of the secrecy that surrounded it, was teaching his wife Parvati the fundamental practices by a river. As he was doing so, a fish (matsya) began to listen with rapt attention. Noticing this, Parvati told her husband, who turned the fish into a man, Matsyendranath, so that he might spread yoga teachings. Matsyendranath is therefore considered the human originator of yoga.

Spend three minutes on this posture. Make sure you always twist to the right first to stimulate the digestive flow; then repeat on the left side.

**1.** Sitting with legs outstretched, bend your right leg up and place your right foot on the outside of the left knee, flat on the floor.

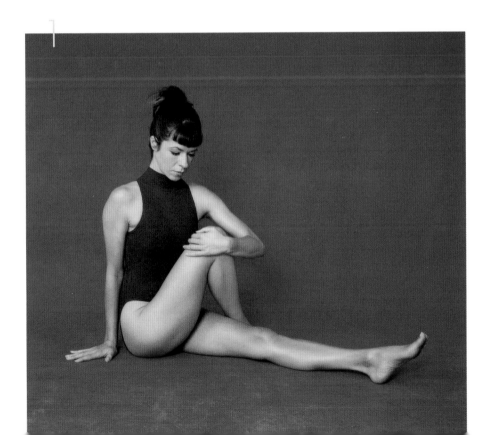

**2.** Place your left hand beside your left hip and, leaning on your left arm, fold your left leg backwards towards the right. Your left heel should now be touching your right buttock.

**3.** Gently, as you breathe, twist your trunk to the right. Aim to catch your right ankle with your left hand. Twist a little more, if possible placing your left arm outside your right thigh, so it acts as a lever for the twist. The right thigh should be pressing the abdomen (picture 2).

**4.** Place your right arm round your back, then straighten your back and open out your chest, breathing deeply and keeping relaxed. As you exhale, progressively deepen the twist, turning your head to the right. Remain in the asana, breathing with awareness, until you are ready to release the posture (picture 3).

### Benefits

This asana massages the spine and abdomen and stretches muscles and nerves in the back, so flooding blood to the heart and lungs. It keeps the spine lithe and free, and is especially good for older people. Another benefit is stimulation of peristalsis which cleanses the colon. According to the Bihar School this asana leads to fruitful introspection!

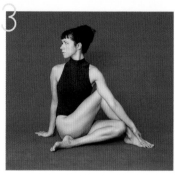

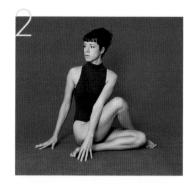

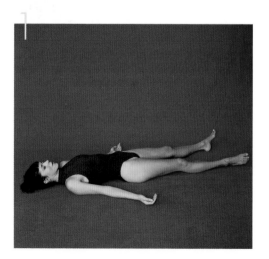

## Savasana

Repeat the Corpse posture for three minutes.

# Nadi Shodana

This alternate nostril breathing sequence involves developing methods for retaining the breath. These methods must be learned with a teacher: do not try to hold your breath for too long too soon. It is interesting to note that the world's free diving champions practise yoga breathing in their training.

You can start by becoming comfortable with the first sequence as described below. Allow ten minutes. (See page 127 for hand positioning.)

## Stage 1

**1.** Sitting comfortably, begin by closing your right nostril with your thumb. Gently inhale and exhale through your left nostril for half the time allocated (picture 1).

**2.** Now close your left nostril with your fourth finger, and slowly inhale and exhale through your right nostril (picture 2).

Practise this every day for a week before moving to stage 2, counting each breath.

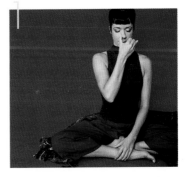

## Stage 2

**1.** Repeat stage one, but every time you inhale or exhale, mentally count 1–2–3 (about one second for each count).

**2.** Now see if you can make the exhalation twice the length of the inhalation – about six counts. Do not strain. One full breath counts as one round.

Aim to practise ten rounds – ten inhalations and ten exhalations, alternating the left and right nostril as described. Practise for two weeks or until it feels comfortable.

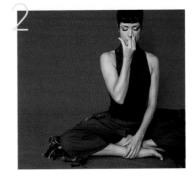

In Tantra, with intensified awareness, every moment of life becomes a meditation.

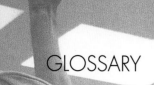

# GLOSSARY

**Acharya**  one who has travelled the way
**Ahimsa**  non-violence
**Angas**  limbs
**Astangas**  eight limbs
**Ardha Baddha Padmottanasana** half-bound lotus (intense), Tree pose
**Ardha Matsyendrasana**  spinal twist
**Ardho Mukha Svanasana**  Downward Dog
**Asana**  Third Limb of yoga; steady posture, balance, poise
**Aum**  three sounds which compose "om", the root mantra
**Ashram**  a house of spiritual retreat
**Artha veda**  the fourth Veda, concerned with medicine and magic
**Ayurveda**  ancient Indian medicine of the Vedas

**Bakasana**  Crow posture
**Bandhas**  energy lock or grip/seal
**Bhagavad Gita**  mystical poem of Krishna, the kernel gem of the Mahabharata
**Bhakti**  heart, surrender; self-denying yoga of devotion
**Bhoga**  enjoyment
**Bhujangasana**  Cobra posture
**Bindu**  creative dot, sacred symbol of the universe, in Tantra equated with sperm

**Chakras**  vortices or wheels of energy; seven psychic energy centres situated along the spine in the subtle body
**Chaturanga Dandasana**  Four-angled Staff pose

**Dhanurasana**  bow
**Dharana**  Sixth Limb of yoga; concentration
**Dhyana**  Seventh Limb of yoga; meditation
**Drishti**  gaze point

**Guna**  attribute, quality; three gunas compose the universe: rajas, sattva and tamas
**Guru**  spiritual teacher, "light dispeller"

**Halasana**  Plough posture
**Hatha**  yoga system using bodily techniques to train the mind

**Ida**  left subtle energy channel which weaves

in a Celtic knot around sushemna, moon energy
**Japa**  constant repetition of a mantra
**Jalandhara**  bandha which closes the glottis at the back of the throat
**Jnana**  yoga of knowledge, self-enquiry

**Karma**  the law of universal cause and effect, action or deeds which, lead one towards or away from bliss; yoga of unconditional service
**Kumbhaka**  breath retention during pranayama
**Kundalini**  latent inner energy, represented by coiled, snake-like, feminine form which normally sleeps but is aroused in Tantric yoga, awakening the creative essence

**Laya**  the awakening of kundalini, absorption of lower grades of energy into higher grades through the subtle body

**Maha bandha**  bandha combining the three main types
**Mandala**  a mystic, circular diagram used for concentrating cosmic and psychic energy
**Mantra**  a Sanskrit syllable, a sacred sound-phrase used to concentrate cosmic or psychic energy; yoga of sound or resonance
**Matsyasana**  Fish posture
**Mayoorasana**  Peacock posture
**Mudra**  seal, gesture to concentrate energy
**Mula bandha**  bandha involving contraction of the perineum

**Nada**  inner sound, the cosmic vibration
**Nadabindu**  seed of the universe as the original first vibration
**Nadi**  energy channel in the subtle body
**Namaste**  prayer position
**Niyama**  Second Limb of yoga; discipline of the body and mind, observances

**Om**  root mantra – the most powerful

**Paddahastasana**  standing forward bend or hands-to-feet posture
**Padamasana**  lotus position
**Padangusthasana**  catching the toes
**Parivrtta Trikonasana**  revolved triangle
**Parsvottanasana**  intense side stretch

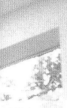

**Paschimottanasana** seated forward bend
**Prana** inner energy or vital air of the subtle body
**Pranayama** Fourth Limb of yoga; the science
of yogic breathing
**Prasarita Padottanasana** expanded leg intense stretch
**Pratyahara** Fifth Limb of yoga; withdrawal of the
senses

**Raja** the royal path or "yoga of kings"
**Rajas** unripeness; one of the three gunas
**Rechaka** exhalation
**Rig veda** the oldest Veda
**Rishi** seer or sage
**Religion** to re-relate; to bridge, to put back together
again

**Sadhana** path
**Saddhu** Hindu holy man, ascetic
**Sahasrara** the top energy centre or chakra at the
crown of the head
**Salabhasana** Locust posture
**Samadhi** Eighth Limb of yoga; final goal of deep
absorption through meditation and concentration
**Samskaras** negative attitudes, mental conditioning
**Sannyasa** final stage of life, cutting the thread of
bondage, renunciation
**Sannyassin** someone who renounces worldly life to
follow a spiritual path
**Sarvangasana** shoulderstand
**Sattva** the highest and purest of the gunas;
state of balance, truth
**Savasana** Corpse posture, relaxation
**Sethubandasana** bridge posture
**Shakti** goddess, the cosmic mother, represents the
feminine principle of universal creative energy central
to Tantric philosophy
**Siddhis** paranormal powers, fruits of yogic practices,
but not their ultimate aim
**Sirsasana** headstand
**Shiva** god of Hinduism, third god of the Hindu trinity,
the destroyer; pure consciousness in Tantra, achieved
in creative union with Shakti
**Subtle body** invisible energy body of nerve channels
existing within the physical body
**Sufis** Islamic mystics who experience
**Suffer** to allow, to bear

a direct link with the divine
**Supta Vajrasana** Recuperation pose
**Suryanamaskar** salutations to the sun
**Sushumna** "she who is gracious", the central energy
channel located within the spine in the subtle body
along which symbolic kundalini energy rises
**Sutra** threads of divine wisdom
**Swami** Indian monks, teachers "who know them-
selves"

**Tadasana** Mountain posture
**Tamas** the power of inertia, lowest of the three gunas
**Tantra** a text embodying Tantric tradition, especially
relating to Shakti power
**Tantrika** practitioner of Tantra
**Tapas** heat, disciplined practice
**Trataka** concentration of vision on a single point
**Trikonasana** triangle, three-pointed posture

**Uddiyana** bandha which seals the lower abdomen
**Ujjayi** deep breathing
**Uttanasana** intense stretch
*Upanishads* spiritual doctrines of ancient Indian
philosophy, concerning the identity of the individual
soul in relation to the universal soul.
**Urdhva Mukha Svanasana** Upward Dog
**Utkatasana** Fierce posture
**Utthita Hasta Padangusthasana** extended hand,
foot and big toe
**Utthita Parsvakonasana** extended side-angle
**Utthita trikonasana** extended triangle

**Vedas** original source books of India, sacred hymns
written in archaic forms of Sanskrit, revealing knowl-
edge of the Aryans, and first references to yoga
**Vedanta** Vedic philosophy imparting
message of oneness
**Vinyasa** breath-synchronized movement
**Virabhadrasana** Warrior pose
**Vishnu** second god of the Hindu triad

**Yama** First Limb of yoga; restraints, rules of conduct
**Yantra** geometrical, symbolic aid to contemplation
**Yoga Nidra** yogic sleep, deep relaxation
**Yogin** male student of yoga
**Yogini** female student of yoga

# FURTHER READING &
# INFORMATION SOURCES

## BOOKS

*The Art of Tantra,* Philip Rawson
(Thames & Hudson, London, 1973)

*Astanga Yoga,* Liz Lark
(Carlton, London, 2000)

*Ashtanga Yoga*
Sri K. Pattabhi Jois,

*Bhagavad Gita,* commentary by
Swami Chidbhavarianda
Sri Ramakrishna Tapovanam
(publication section),
Tirupparaitturai – 639 115,
Tiruchirappalli Dt, Tamil Nadu,
(1986)

*Bliss Divine, Spiritual Essays,*
Swami Sivananda
Divine Life Society,
P.O. Shivanandanagar 249 1921993,
India (1997)

*The Heart of Yoga, Developing a
personal practice,*
T.K.V. Desikachar, Inner Traditions, 1
Park Street, Rochester Vermont
05767, U.S.A (www.gotoit.com),1995

*How to Know God: The Yoga
Aphorisms of Patanjali,*
commentary by Swami
Prabhavananda and Christopher
Isherwood (Vedanta Press, 1953)

*Introduction to Tantra – A Vision
of Totality,*
Lama Yeshe,
(Wisdom Publications, Boston, 1987)

*Moola Bandha,*
The Master Key,
Chela Buddhananda,
Bihar School of Yoga, India, 1978

*Owning Your Own Shadow,*
Robert A Johnson
(Harper, San Francisco, 1991)

*Ravi Shankar, An Autobiography,*
edited by George Harrison,
Genesis Publications Ltd,
2 Jenner Road, Guildford,
Surrey GU1 3PL, England/
Element, Shaftesbury,
Dorset SP7 8BP, England,
1997/1999

*Return to the Centre,*
Bede Griffiths
(Fount paperbacks, 1978)

*The Sivananda Training Manual,*
Sivananda Yoga Vedanta Centre,
51 Felsham Road, London
SW15 1AZ,
England (1991)

*A Systematic Course in The Ancient
Tantric Techniques of Yoga and Kriya,*
Swami Satyananda Saraswati,
Bihar School of Yoga,
Bihar, India (1981)

*Tantra, The Path of Ecstasy,*
Georg Feuerstein,
(Shambhala, India, 1998)

*The Tantric Way,*
Ajit Mookerjee and Madhu Khanna,
(Thames & Hudson, London, 1977)

*Tantra Yoga,* Nik Douglas,
Munshiram Manoharlal,
New Delhi, India (1971)

*Yoga Asanas,*
Divine Life Society,
P.O. Shivanandanagar 249 1921993,
U. P. , Himalayas, India, 1993

*Yoga for Beginners,*
Liz Lark and Mark Ansari,
(Newleaf, UK, 1998)

*Yoga Mala,*
Yogasana Visharada Vedanta
Vidvan,
Sri K. Pattabhi Jois,
(Eddie Stern/Patanjali Yogashala,
New York, 1999)

*Yoga Self-Taught,*
Andrei Van Lysbeth,
(Samuel Weiser Inc, York Beach,
Maine, USA, 1999)

*The Yoga Tradition,*
Hohm Press, P.O. Box 2501,
Prescott, Arizona 86302, USA

*From Here to Nirvana: Yoga Journal's
Guide to Spiritual India,* Anne
Cushman and Jerry Jones
(Yoga Journal, USA)

*Light on Yoga: Yogi Dipika,*
B. K. S. Iyengar
(Schocken Books, USA, 1995)

*The Healing Path of Yoga,*
Nischala Devi
(Three Rivers Press, USA, 2000)

*Yoga Mind, Body and Spirit: A
Return to Wholeness,* Donna Farhi
(Henry Holt, USA, 2000)

## JOURNALS
*Yoga & Health,*
Yoga Today Ltd,
Sussex, England,
tel +44 (0) 1273 563111

*Yoga Journal*
+1-800-1-DO-YOGA

## VIDEOS

*Yoga: The Ultimate Freedom*,
B.K.S. Iyengar, Yogaware,
Ann Arbor,
Michigan, Canada,
tel (734) 663688191976

*Yoga Masterclass with B.K.S.
Iyengar*, Iyengar Institute (see
below)

*Yoga Alignment and Form* with
John Friend
(90 minutes $19.95)

*Yoga Zone*
Beginners boxed set
(4 tapes – $39.95)

## YOGA CENTRES AND SCHOOLS

**Astanga Yoga,**
Gingi Lee & Liz Lark
Sangam
80b Battersea Rise,
London SW11 1EH,
England

**Bihar School of Yoga,**
Mungar, Bihar, 811 201, India

**British Wheel of Yoga,**
1 Hamilton Place,
Boston Road, Sleaford,
Lincs NG34 7ES, England

**Iyengar Institute,**
223 Randolph Avenue,
Maida Vale,
London, England W9 1NL,
www.iyi.org.uk

**Satyananda Yoga Centre,**
UK, fax +44 (0) 208 6754080,
www.yoga.freeuk.com

**Satyananda Yoga Centre,**
70 Thurleigh Road,
London SW12 8UD, England

**Sivananda Ashram Yoga Camp,**
8th Ave, Val Morin,
Quebec, Canada JOT 2RO

**Sivananda Yoga Vedanta Centre,**
51 Felsham Rd,
London SW15 1AZ, England,
www.SivanandaYoga.org

**Viniyoga Britain,**
tel/fax 44 (0) 1293 536664

**Ruth White Yoga Centre,**
Church Farm House,
Spring Close Lane,
Cheam, Surrey SM3 8PU, England

**Sangam Yoga Centre**
Gingi Lee & Liz Lark
80b Battersea Rise,
London SW11 1EH, England

**Yoga Biomedical Trust,**
P.O. Box 140,
Cambridge BD4 3SY, England

**Yoga Therapy Centre,**
Royal Homeopathic Hospital
Trust, 60 Great Ormond Street,
London WC1N 3HR, England

**Jivamukti Yoga Center Inc.**
404 Lafayette Street #3
New York, NY, USA
+1-212-353-0214

**Sivananda Yoga Center**
1246 West Bryn Mawr Avenue,
Chicago, IL, USA
+1-773-878-7771

**B. K. S. Iyengar Yoga School**
321 Divisadero Street,
San Francisco, CA, USA
+1-415-626-8441

## USEFUL WEBSITES

www.booknotes.com/hohm
www.sourcetantra.com
www.tantra.com
www.viniyoga.co.uk
www.lizlark.com

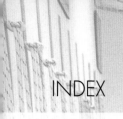

# INDEX

## Aknowledgements

Thank you to all who contributed to this book: Gill Lloyd and Andrew Payne; Swami Pragyamurti and grand-son; Ruth White; Jean Hall; Gingi Lee; Matthew Vollmer; Dominic Parks; Catriona Brokenshire; Panni, Ganga and Kailash Bharti; Sabel Thierri and Jennifer Dale; Miles Taylor; Andrea Durrant; Bob Walters; Justine Hardy; Anya Evans; Lisskulla Junglist; Ivengar Yoga Institute and students, Maida Vale; Sangam Yoga Centre and students, Battersea and Tri Yoga, Primrose Hill. A special thank you also to Clare Park for her wonderful photography and all her help.

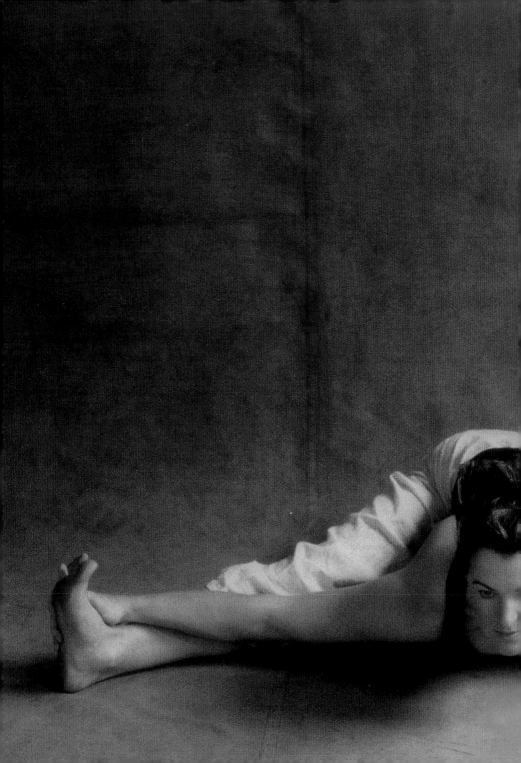

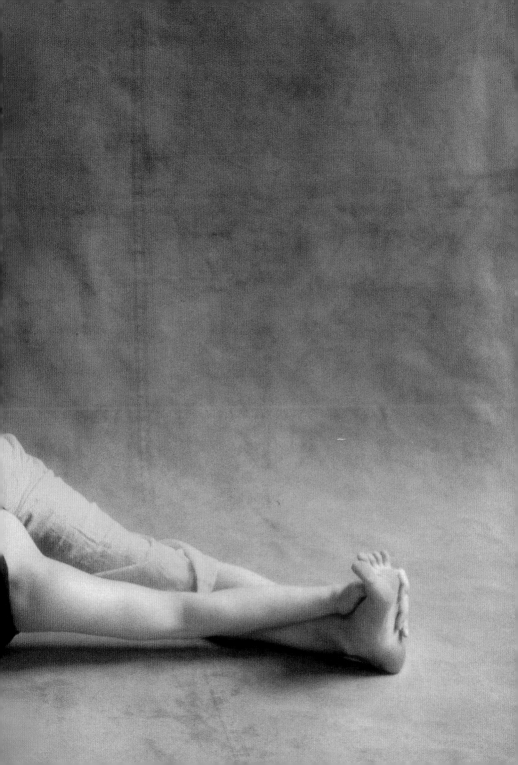

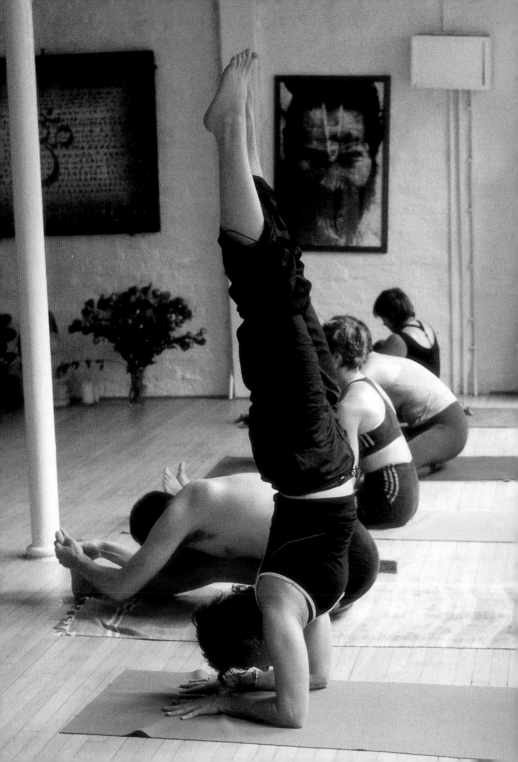

<< To see a **world** in a grain of sand

and a heaven in a **wild flower**

hold **infinity** in the palm of your hand

and **eternity** in an hour. >>

WILLIAM BLAKE

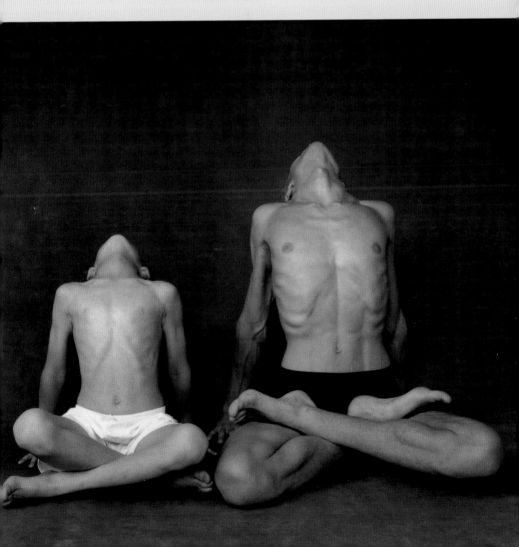

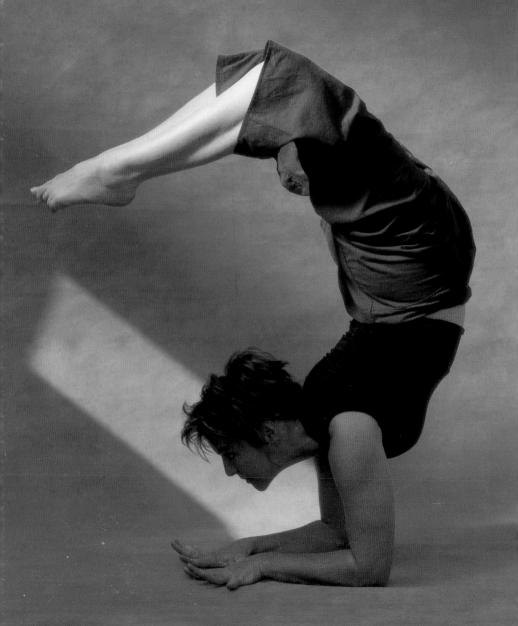

" I inhabit my soul. " WALT WHITMAN